the
vegan
athlete's
cookbook

the vegan athlete's cookbook

Protein-rich recipes to train, recover and perform

ANITA BEAN

BLOOMSBURY SPORT

LONDON · OXFORD · NEW YORK · NEW DELHI · SYDNEY

BLOOMSBURY SPORT
Bloomsbury Publishing Plc
50 Bedford Square, London, WC1B 3DP, UK
29 Earlsfort Terrace, Dublin 2, Ireland

BLOOMSBURY, BLOOMSBURY SPORT and the Diana logo
are trademarks of Bloomsbury Publishing Plc

First published in Great Britain 2021

The information contained in this book is provided by way of
general guidance in relation to the specific subject matters
addressed herein, but it is not a substitute for specialist
dietary advice. It should not be relied on for medical,
health-care, pharmaceutical or other professional advice on
specific dietary or health needs. This book is sold with the
understanding that the author and publisher are not engaged
in rendering medical, health or any other kind of personal or
professional services. The reader should consult a competent
medical or health professional before adopting any of the
suggestions in this book or drawing inferences from it.

The author and publisher specifically disclaim, as far as the
law allows, any responsibility from any liability, loss or risk
(personal or otherwise) which is incurred as a consequence,
directly or indirectly, of the use and applications of any of
the contents of this book. If you are on medication of any
description, please consult your doctor or health
professional before embarking on any fast or diet.

Bloomsbury Publishing Plc does not have any control
over, or responsibility for, any third-party websites
referred to or in this book. All internet addresses given
in this book were correct at the time of going to press.
The author and publisher regret any inconvenience
caused if addresses have changed or sites have ceased
to exist, but can accept no responsibility for any
such changes

A catalogue record for this book is available from the
British Library

Library of Congress Cataloguing-in-Publication data
has been applied for

ISBN: PB: 978-1-4729-8429-6;
      ePub: 978-1-4729-8428-9;
      ePDF: 978-1-4729-8427-2

10 9 8 7 6 5 4 3 2 1

Designed by Austin Taylor
Typeset in Aestetico and Laca
Printed and bound in India by Replika Press Pvt. Ltd.

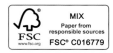

To find out more about our authors and books visit
www.bloomsbury.com and sign up for our newsletters

Contents

Introduction

Welcome to my fourth sports nutrition cookbook, in which I aim to show you how incredibly tasty and nutritious vegan cooking can be.

Writing a solely vegan book for athletes has been a dream of mine since I wrote *The Vegetarian Athlete's Cookbook* (Bloomsbury Sport, 2016). Many of you have told me how much you enjoyed the vegan recipes and it is clear that more and more of you are adopting increasingly meat- and dairy-free diets. So, I have created a brand-new collection of delicious vegan recipes, which are packed with all the nutrients you need to train, perform and recover. In addition, this book provides evidence-based advice on how to optimise your performance on a vegan diet. It features my Vegan Athlete's Plate, an easy tool to help you build a balanced diet and fuel your workouts on easy, moderate and hard training days.

Until relatively recently, veganism was considered faddy, unhealthy and restrictive. It certainly held little appeal for athletes who had long believed that animal products were essential for athletic performance. Certainly, when I was competing as a vegetarian bodybuilder in the nineties, the idea that you could compete successfully without eating meat was unheard of. I was always asked where I was getting my protein from, which is understandable as meat has long been synonymous with strength. Nonetheless, I managed to prove the doubters wrong when I won the British Bodybuilding Championships and finished in the top 10 at the World Championships. I retired from competition but have maintained a daily exercise habit either with weight training, road cycling, yoga, running or hiking.

Thankfully, attitudes have changed since the nineties and I have seen a huge rise in interest in vegan diets among athletes in my practice – including male athletes – which is a big departure from the social stereotype of a meat-eating athlete. Much of this interest in vegan diets has been fuelled by a shifting awareness of the health, performance and environmental impacts of a vegan diet (which are covered in Chapter 2, *see* pp. 14–20).

WHAT IS A VEGAN DIET?

A vegan diet is one that excludes all animal products, including meat, fish, poultry, dairy products, eggs and honey. Most vegans also avoid wearing animal-derived materials such as fur, leather, silk and wool and using household products and cosmetics containing animal-derived ingredients. The Vegan Society defines veganism as a way of living which seeks to exclude, as far as is possible and practicable, all forms of exploitation of, and cruelty to, animals for food, clothing or any other purpose. You may have heard the term 'plant-based', which is sometimes used interchangeably with 'vegan' but sometimes with a vegetarian, pescatarian (includes fish), or flexitarian diet that still includes small amounts of animal products. In fact, there is no universally agreed definition of the term, which in my view renders it rather meaningless. So, I have used the term 'vegan' throughout this book.

Many people, including myself, love animals and don't want to see them suffer, so choosing a more ethical and compassionate way of eating makes perfect sense. Additionally, vegan campaigns such as Veganuary and Netflix documentaries, such as *The Game Changers*, have helped to get a powerful message out there: that you don't need to eat animal products to perform well in sport. As a result, an increasing number of world-class athletes from many different sports, including ultra-endurance and endurance, strength, power and team sports, have switched to a vegan diet.

Outside the world of sport, vegan diets have also grown in popularity. The number of vegans in the UK has quadrupled between 2014 and 2019 to more than 600,000, a number that's likely to grow substantially in the coming years.[1] According to a poll carried out on behalf of Waitrose & Partners, one in eight (13 per cent) people now identify as vegan or vegetarian and a further 21 per cent as flexitarian (mostly vegetarian with occasional meat).[2] Six per cent of the US population and about 10 per cent of Europeans are vegetarian and vegan.[3,4] It is clear that veganism is on the rise.

Veganism does not have to be all or nothing, though. Simply going vegan one day a week or substituting more vegan meals for meat in your weekday or weekend routine is a great place to start and means you will be getting more plant nutrients that will protect against chronic lifestyle-related illnesses, support your athletic performance and promote recovery. You can be a part-time vegan if you want and then decide whether you adopt this way of eating long-term.

What makes this book different from other vegan cookbooks is its focus on performance. Every recipe has been created to provide a high level of nutrients that will fuel your workouts and promote recovery. Uniquely, all the main meal recipes in this book supply at least 20 g protein per serving, which is the optimal amount needed for muscle recovery.

What else can you expect in this book? In Chapter 1, you will find popular myths about vegan diets debunked and in Chapter 4, a deeper dive into the question of where vegans can get their protein. And if you want to know exactly what a vegan diet can do for you, then head to Chapter 2, which highlights the health, performance and environmental advantages of this way of eating. All of this information is backed up by published studies and I have provided references at the end of the book so that you can read more about them.

While a well-planned vegan diet can be an extremely healthy way of eating, I am also aware that some people look to veganism as a way of losing weight. For non-athletes, this can be an effective strategy, but if you exercise regularly then you do need to ensure you eat enough to fuel your training without compromising your health. An overly restricted vegan diet can quickly result in energy deficiency, health problems and reduced performance. In Chapter 3, I flag up the early warning signs to watch out for and explain how you can ensure you avoid these pitfalls.

Of course, having the freedom to choose to eat a varied and healthy diet is a privilege. And while we are free to choose to eat a vegan diet, we should not cast judgement on other people's food choices nor allow our dietary beliefs to set us apart from other people. Everyone is entitled to choose a diet that best fits their ethics, philosophy, tastes, special dietary requirements and finances.

I am a strong believer that vegan food should not be boring and in this book I hope to prove that it can be exciting and incredibly tasty. Eating is one of life's great pleasures and we should never feel guilty for enjoying our food or spending time, money and effort in attaining it. I love making and eating vegan food and I hope that the recipes in this book will inspire you to develop a passion for vegan food, too.

Enjoy!

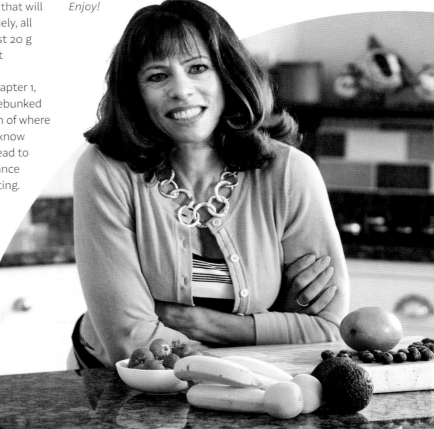

PART 1

Vegan sports nutrition

1

Vegan myths

Although vegan diets have come a long way in last few years, there remain many myths and misconceptions surrounding them, particularly when it comes to athletic performance. Naysayers are always quick to cite a story of someone who became unwell on a vegan diet before switching back to eating animal products. But this is not a valid argument against vegan diets.

Such anecdotes are invariably devoid of context or nuance. If you cut out animal products without replacing them with suitable alternatives or adopt a poorly planned vegan diet with the sole aim of weight loss, then you will likely develop health problems. But you cannot say that all vegan diets are harmful or that animal products are necessary for health.

People are often quick to judge and criticise vegans for their dietary choices. Such objections usually come in the guise of health and nutritional concerns – which I will address in this chapter – but many of these are unfounded and not supported by science. Such beliefs about the negative health consequences of vegan diets are often born out of prejudice or simply a lack of knowledge and education about nutrition. It's easy to be sceptical or even critical of vegan diets if you do not have the facts and evidence. But there are of course also legitimate pitfalls with vegan diets, which I address in Chapter 3 (*see* pp. 21–30). If you are worried about whether a vegan diet can provide you with enough nutrients to support your training goals, then this chapter will help to put your mind at rest.

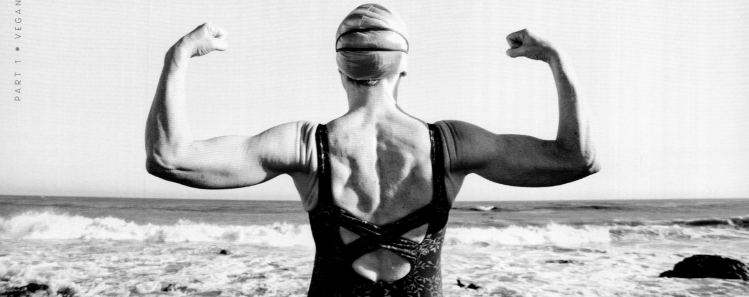

MYTH 1 Vegans cannot get enough protein

This is probably the biggest myth about vegan diets. On the contrary, a review of studies published in the journal *Nutrients* in 2019 concluded that there is no evidence of protein deficiency among vegetarians and vegans in Western countries.[1] Most people, whether vegan or not, get more than enough protein and have little difficulty meeting the recommended intake. The EPIC-Oxford study of 40,000 people found that while the average protein intake of vegans (0.99 g/kg body weight/day) was less than that of non-vegans (1.28 g/kg of body weight/day), it still exceeded the recommended daily intake (0.75 g/kg of body weight/day).[2] According to the Academy of Nutrition and Dietetics, vegan diets typically meet or exceed recommended protein intakes when energy needs are also met.[3] This view is endorsed by the British Dietetic Association, which states that 'well-planned plant-based diets can support healthy living at every age and life-stage'.[4] While athletes need more protein than the general population, provided you are consuming enough energy (calories) to meet your fuel requirements *and* you are eating a wide variety of plant-based protein foods, such as soya products, beans, lentils, grains, nuts and seeds during the course of the day, then it is very likely that you are getting all the protein you need.

MYTH 2 You cannot build muscle on a vegan diet

Many people associate muscle almost exclusively with meat and believe therefore that animal proteins are essential for building muscle. This is false as studies have shown that provided you consume enough protein it does not matter whether it comes from animals or plants.[5] Researchers have also shown that plant proteins, such as soya, and animal proteins, such as whey, produce similar gains in strength and muscle mass following resistance training.[6] Although athletes generally need more protein than the general population, it is not difficult to get enough from plant sources – even if you are a heavyweight bodybuilder. The key is

1 to eat plant proteins in sufficient quantity – 20 g (or 0.25 g/kg of body weight) of protein per meal is thought to be optimal (*see* p. 32).[7] Aim to get this from whole foods wherever possible, otherwise include protein supplements if you need to (*see* p. 37).
2 to ensure you eat a variety of different plant proteins over the course of the day.
3 to include plant foods rich in the amino acid leucine (e.g. soya products, beans and lentils), which is an important trigger for the process of muscle building.

So, with a bit of planning, it is easy to supply the body with more than enough quality protein to build and maintain muscle on a vegan diet. As a bonus, you will also get plenty of other nutrients such as carbohydrate, unsaturated fat, vitamins, minerals, phytonutrients (plant nutrients that confer health benefits) and fibre that you will not find in animal foods.

MYTH 3 Plant proteins are incomplete

The idea that plant proteins are incomplete or 'missing' specific amino acids is false. All plant foods contain all 20 amino acids, including the nine essential amino acids (EAA, *see* p. 34), albeit some at low levels – but they do not lack any.[1,8,9] A more accurate statement would be that the amino acid profile in plant foods is less optimal for our body's needs than animal foods. For example, lysine is present in relatively low amounts in grains and, similarly, methionine is proportionally slightly lower in beans and lentils. This would only be a problem if you ate only grains or beans every day but since most people eat a mixture of plant proteins, this means you can easily get all 20 amino acids to cover your requirements.

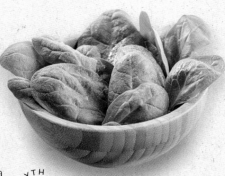

MYTH 4 You need to combine plant proteins at each meal

This myth was inadvertently popularised in the book, *Diet for a Small Planet*, by Frances Moore Lappé in 1971.[10] It promoted the idea of 'protein combining', i.e. that we need to eat a combination of certain plant foods *at the same time* in order to get all of the essential amino acids (EAAs). The theory has since been proved incorrect and the author later retracted her statement in a revised edition of the book published in 1981. She wrote that in trying to combat one myth, that meat is the only way to get high-quality protein, she had created a second one – the myth of the need for protein combining.

Plant proteins do not need to be combined within a single meal. Studies have shown that our bodies pool the amino acids we need as we eat them over a 24-hour period and we draw on this pool and use them as needed.[11] What matters most is our total intake of amino acids over the course of the day. As long as we consume enough EAAs throughout the day and we are meeting our energy (calorie) requirements, then our body will get all it needs over time.

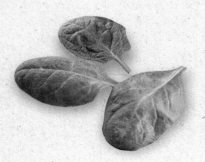

MYTH 5 A vegan diet will lack iron

Iron deficiency is more likely to occur as a result of inadequate absorption or excessive loss through menstruation rather than a low dietary intake. Studies show that vegans are no more susceptible to iron deficiency than non-vegans.

Many people believe that meat is the only real source of iron but, in fact, iron is found in a wide variety of plant foods, including beans, lentils, leafy green vegetables, nuts and seeds (*see* p. 26). Although iron is not as readily absorbed from plants as meat, the body adjusts absorption according to its iron needs. For example, if your iron levels fall, then the body will absorb more from your food. In other words, it is not about how much iron is in your food, but how well you absorb it.

Eating foods rich in in vitamin C (most fruit or vegetables) at the same time as iron-rich foods greatly improves iron absorption. Citric acid (also found naturally in fruit and vegetables) also promotes iron absorption. So, if you eat a varied diet that includes a wide variety of iron sources, then you are no more at risk of iron deficiency than a meat eater.

MYTH 6 You will have less energy

Most people actually have more energy after switching to a vegan diet. This is likely because cutting out meat and eating instead more beans, lentils, nuts, fruit and vegetables results in a higher intake of vitamins, minerals and phytonutrients, which strengthens your immune system. If your energy levels do drop, you are probably not matching your calories to your training. This can sometimes happen in endurance athletes during periods of heavy training when energy demands are high. It is all down to a concept called low energy availability (LEA) and happens when there is a mismatch between your energy intake and the energy requirements of your training programme (*see* p. 24). Vegan diets tend to be higher in fibre, more filling and have a lower energy (calorie) density than non-vegan diets. While this may be advantageous for people wishing to lose weight, it can also make it difficult for some athletes to meet their energy needs. However, LEA is not a unique feature of vegan diets – it can also happen with non-vegan diets. Chapter 3 shows you how to avoid the nutritional pitfalls of vegan diets and ensure you get enough energy.

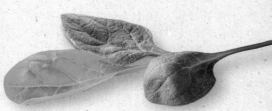

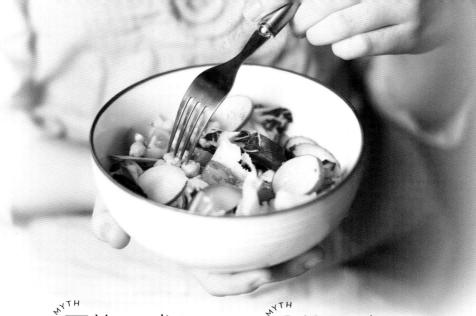

MYTH 9 Soya is harmful

There is no evidence to support this belief. A 2019 review of hundreds of studies linked soya to lower rates of heart disease, certain cancers and lower blood cholesterol and found that it may help relieve hot flushes during the menopause.[13] Similarly, fears about soya causing breast cancer in women are unfounded. They stem from soya's content of isoflavones (phytoestrogens), which have a similar structure to the body's own oestrogen, high levels of which have been linked to an increased risk of breast cancer. However, soya isoflavones have much weaker effects in the body (if at all) and there is no evidence that they increase the risk of breast cancer.[14] Reassuringly, a number of large studies have concluded that diets high in traditional soya foods such as tofu, tempeh, edamame, miso and soya milk alternative are, in fact, *protective* against breast cancer and may also prevent breast cancer recurrence and increase survival rate.[15] In one study of more than 73,000 Chinese women, researchers found that higher intakes of soya were associated with a reduced risk of breast cancer.[16] Soya foods are excellent sources of protein, providing high amounts of all nine essential amino acids, making them valuable foods for vegan athletes. They are also a good source of unsaturated fats, fibre, B vitamins, iron and calcium.

MYTH 7 Vegan diets leave you hungry

If you are hungry on a vegan diet, then you are doing something wrong – namely, not eating enough whole foods or not eating enough protein. Whole foods, such as beans, lentils, whole grains, fruit, vegetables, nuts and seeds, are full of fibre, which literally keeps you full for longer and stabilises blood sugar levels to prevent hunger soon after eating. It also helps to satisfy your hunger by slowing down the rate that foods pass through your digestive system. Getting enough protein is important, too, as it helps to promote satiety and keeps you full longer. So, if you are relying more on heavily processed foods than whole foods or not including sufficient protein in each meal, then you will not be getting the protein and fibre you need to feel full and satisfied.

MYTH 8 Vegan diets make you more prone to illness

Quite the reverse, a well-planned vegan diet can actively increase your resistance to illness and infection – provided you are consuming enough energy (calories) and focusing on whole foods such as beans, lentils, grains, fruit, vegetables, nuts and seeds. All of these foods are rich in antioxidant nutrients and phytonutrients (particularly polyphenols, *see* p. 16) that help foster a healthy gut microbiome (*see* p. 17) and strengthen your immune defences. Indeed, studies have shown that vegans have improved immune cell activity and lower levels of inflammatory markers, all of which translate into greater protection against illness.[12] The bottom line is that every athlete, vegan or not, needs to ensure that they fuel adequately for their sport and focus on the nutritional quality of their diet in order to prevent illness.

2

The vegan advantage: health, performance and the environment

A vegan diet – or at least including more vegan meals in your diet – can offer numerous advantages to athletes at every level. A growing body of scientific evidence over the last 50 years suggests that diets centred around plants have clear health advantages over those based on animal foods.[1] They are associated with a longer life span, lower risk of heart disease, certain cancers and other chronic diseases.

Although our knowledge is far from complete, it is becoming increasingly clear that a vegan diet can also support sports performance and that athletes at all levels can gain a performance advantage from eating this way. Avoiding animal products also benefits the environment and goes a long way towards reducing climate change and cutting your carbon footprint. This chapter provides a scientific round-up of the evidence so you can make your own mind up.

The health advantage

According to the Academy of Nutrition and Dietetics, the world's largest professional organisation for registered dietitians and nutritionists, well-planned vegan (and vegetarian) diets are healthy, nutritionally adequate, match dietary guidelines and meet current recommended intakes, provide health benefits for the prevention and treatment of certain diseases and are appropriate for people of all ages, as well as for athletes.[2] Vegan diets have also been endorsed by the British Dietetic Association as healthy for all people of all ages.[3]

Although it is difficult to determine cause and effect when it comes to food and disease, what we do know is that people who eat more plants in their diet tend to have lower overall risk of diseases, including obesity, high blood pressure (hypertension), type 2 diabetes, certain cancers, and a consistently lower risk of death due to heart disease, compared to those who eat a typical Western diet

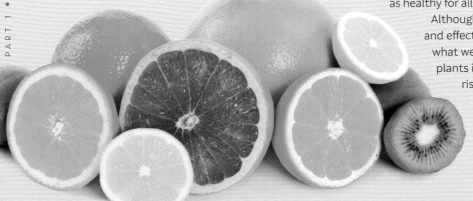

high in refined carbohydrates, sugar and heavily-processed foods.[4, 5, 6, 7, 8] Here is a summary of the evidence:

• An analysis of three long-term studies of Seventh-day Adventists in Loma Linda, California, USA (a religious denomination who lead a conservative lifestyle) found that those eating a vegetarian or vegan diet lived longer and had lower risk of heart disease, stroke and certain cancers than those who ate meat.[9] Vegans in particular were also less likely to develop obesity, hypertension, type-2 diabetes or cardiovascular disease risk.

• An analysis of five prospective studies published in the *American Journal of Clinical Nutrition* in 1999 found that vegans had a 26 per cent lower risk of death from heart disease than non-vegans, largely due to their lower cholesterol levels[10]

• A review of large-scale prospective studies showed that colorectal cancer is more common among people who eat lots of red meat and processed meat. Overall, eating red and processed meat increases colorectal cancer by 20–30 per cent[11]

• The Global Burden of Disease study, the most comprehensive worldwide observational epidemiological study to date and published in *The Lancet* in 2019, concluded that diets low in whole grains, fruit, vegetables, nuts and seeds are the biggest dietary risk factors for premature death[12]

• A study published in the *Journal of the American Medical Association* in 2019 showed that substituting plant protein for red meat protein can lower total, cancer-related and cardiovascular disease-related mortality[13]

• A review of studies published in 2019 concluded that vegan and vegetarian diets can help protect against chronic metabolic diseases and certain cancers, with links found between plant protein intake and healthier markers of heart health, management of type 2 diabetes and improved weight management[14]

IS MEAT BAD FOR YOU?

A 2018 report by the World Cancer Research Fund (WCRF) concluded that there is strong evidence that consumption of either red or processed meats are both causes of colorectal cancer.[19] Processed meat is meat that has been salted, cured, fermented, smoked or blended to make ham, bacon, beef jerky, corned beef, salami, pepperoni or hot dogs. It has also been linked to other cancers, including breast, pancreas and prostate. The WCRF recommend cutting out processed meat altogether and no more than 350–500 g unprocessed red meat a week. The increased cancer risk among those who eat meat may be due to a number of factors, including a lack of fibre, a lower intake of plant foods, less exercise, or to certain chemicals found in the meat itself. One theory is that cooking meat at high temperatures (e.g. during frying, grilling or barbecuing) produces chemicals called heterocyclic amines (HCAs) and polycyclic aromatic hydrocarbons (PAH) and these may trigger cancer. In addition, iron found naturally in red meat is broken down to form carcinogenic (cancer-causing) compounds in the bowel. Another theory is that N-nitroso compounds, potent cancer-carcinogens, are formed when meat is processed by smoking, curing or salting, or by the addition of nitrites or nitrates.

• A study published in the *European Journal of Clinical Nutrition* found that substituting soya, beans and lentils for red meat significantly improved fasting blood glucose levels, insulin, triglycerides and LDL-cholesterol in people with type 2 diabetes[15]

• A comprehensive analysis of 96 previous studies at the University of Florence, Italy, found that people eating a vegan diet had a 15 per cent lower risk of cancer. They also had significantly lower body weights and total and LDL-cholesterol levels than those who ate meat[16]

• The European Prospective Investigation into Cancer and Nutrition (EPIC)-Oxford study involving 45,000 British people found that vegans and vegetarians have a 32 per cent lower risk of heart disease than omnivores (meat-eaters), which the researchers attribute to the lower body mass index, blood pressure and blood cholesterol measured in this group[17]

• A study by a German researcher published in 1993 showed that the longevity and cancer-protective benefits increase with time. Those who ate a vegetarian diet for 20 years or more had a lower risk of dying early and chronic disease than those who had been vegetarian for fewer years, as well as those who ate meat[18]

The performance advantage

The American College of Sports Medicine states that 'well-planned vegetarian and vegan diets appear to successfully and effectively support parameters that influence athletic performance'.[20] But the idea that a diet centred on plants supports sports performance is certainly not new. In Roman times, the gladiators – who were reputed to be the best fighters in the world – ate a mainly vegetarian diet to increase their stamina and strength.[21] Nowadays, we are seeing more and more world-class athletes from virtually every sport shunning animal products in favour of a vegetarian or vegan diet. They provide compelling anecdotal evidence that you can compete at a high-level without eating animal products. Thanks to the growing number of athletes from virtually every sport, the old image of a weak vegan athlete has been buried. Even Hollywood's Arnold Schwarzenegger – a former bodybuilder – has joined the ranks of converts. Athletes claim to have had increased energy, faster recovery, less illness and fewer injuries since turning vegan. Vegan eating has now become not only acceptable among athletes, but even desirable. One thing is certain – we do not need to eat animal products to be healthy or perform in sport.

It is clear that athletes can train and compete at a high level on a well-planned, nutrient-rich, whole-food vegan diet. Although fewer studies have looked directly at the effects of a vegan or vegetarian diet on performance, they all provide compelling evidence that excluding animal products does not put you at a *disadvantage* when it comes to fitness or performance:

- A review of studies by Canadian researchers in 2004 concluded that well-planned vegan and vegetarian diets can support athletic performance.[22] Provided protein intakes are adequate to meet needs for total nitrogen and the essential amino acids, plant and animal protein sources can provide equivalent support to athletic training and performance

- In a German study published in 1994, vegetarian and non-vegetarian German runners taking part in a 1000-km race over 20 days had all their food provided to ensure they all received the same amount of energy (calories), carbohydrate, fat and protein.[23] There was no difference in finishing times between the two groups, suggesting that a vegetarian diet does not adversely affect running performance
- A review of eight previous studies by Australian researchers in 2016 found no differences in performance between vegans, vegetarians and omnivores, and concluded that well-planned and varied vegetarian or vegan diets neither hinder nor improve performance in athletes[24]
- A study of endurance athletes at Arizona State University in 2016 found that vegetarian athletes had similar strength and greater cardiorespiratory fitness than those who ate meat and concluded that a vegetarian diet may even be advantageous for supporting aerobic fitness in athletes[25]
- A study of runners following a vegan, vegetarian or meat-based diet published in the *Journal of the International Society of Sports Nutrition* in 2019 found no difference in their maximal power output and exercise capacity.[26] They concluded that a vegan diet could support athletic performance in runners

Why is a vegan diet good for your health and performance?

Many of the health and performance advantages of a vegan diet are likely due to the higher consumption of nutrients found in plant foods. Beans, lentils and peas, for example, provide protein, complex carbohydrates, soluble and insoluble fibre, B vitamins, magnesium, iron, zinc and potassium. Nuts and seeds provide unsaturated fats, fibre and protein, along with vitamin E, iron, zinc and phytonutrients. Fruit and vegetables contain a high level of vitamin C, folate and beta-carotene. Plant foods are also rich in polyphenols, which help support the immune system and benefit our health in many other ways. The EPIC-Oxford study, one of the largest studies of vegans in the world, showed that vegans had higher intakes of fibre, magnesium, iron, folic acid, thiamine and vitamins C and E than vegetarians or omnivores.[27] In other words, it's not necessarily the absence of animal products that's helping vegans perform and recover better, rather their higher intake of fibre and plant nutrients (which help combat inflammation) and lower intake of saturated fat and extrinsic (added) sugars (which provoke inflammation). However, it is possible that other lifestyle factors may also play a role: vegans generally tend to exercise more and weigh less, and are less likely to smoke and drink excessive alcohol, all of which may account for some of the reduction in disease risk.

The gut connection

Plant foods are also thought to influence your health and performance via their positive effect on your gut microbiota, the trillions of microbes (bacteria, yeast, fungi and viruses) that live in your digestive tract. The fibre and polyphenols that they contain feed your 'good' gut microbes, helping them grow and multiply. As they do so, they produce beneficial substances, including vitamins (namely B vitamins and vitamin K) and short-chain fatty acids (acetate, propionate and butyrate) that provide fuel for your intestinal, liver and muscle cells, and have a huge impact on many aspects of your health, including immunity and sporting performance and recovery.

A review of studies published in 2020 concluded that having a diverse microbiota – a wide array of different microbial species – may have bigger performance benefits.[28] Although the exact mechanisms are not fully understood, it is likely that there are several indirect effects that result in a performance-boosting effect. These include increased immunity, less oxidative stress (*see box* p. 18) and lower inflammation (*see box* p. 19), all key factors necessary for performance and muscle recovery after exercise.[29, 30] With better immunity, you are less likely to suffer illnesses and gut problems that can hamper your training (*see* p. 19). And with less oxidative stress and lower inflammation, you will have less muscle damage and faster recovery. Additionally, the short-chain fatty acids produced by 'good' gut microbes help regulate energy metabolism, appetite hormones and body composition.

A meta-analysis of studies found that people who consumed a vegetarian or vegan diet for at least two years had lower levels of inflammation (as measured by lower blood levels of C-reactive protein) than those who ate meat, suggesting such diets have an anti-inflammatory effect on the body.[31] A 2019 review of studies points to the benefits of foods rich in anthocyanins (a subclass of polyphenols found in fruit and vegetables) for increasing the population of beneficial gut microbes, while at the same time inhibiting the harmful species.[32]

In other words, a healthy gut microbiota is critical for optimal performance and recovery, as well as health. A vegan diet results in a proliferation of healthy microbe species, a healthier gut microbiota, less inflammation in the body and a more favourable body composition, all of which roughly translates into better athletic performance.

How can you improve your gut health?

Improving your gut health by switching to a vegan diet will increase the diversity of your gut microbes, which in turn may improve your overall health, sports performance and post-exercise recovery. A study at Harvard University showed that you can achieve this within as little as five days.[33]

The best way to boost the diversity of your gut microbes – and gain a performance advantage – is to eat a wide range of plant foods rich in fibre, polyphenols and prebiotics. These provide food for your 'good' gut microbes so they can grow. There are many types of fibre and the more types you eat, the greater the benefit. The

American Gut Project, a large-scale study that analysed microbiome samples from more than 10,000 individuals, showed that people who eat around 30 different plants each week have much greater microbial diversity than those who eat just 10.[34]

● **Plant-based foods** – Try to get as many different kinds of fruit, vegetables, whole grains, beans, lentils, nuts and seeds in your diet as possible. Variety is key because each contains different nutrients that the gut microbes thrive on

WHAT IS OXIDATIVE STRESS?

Oxidative stress occurs during intense exercise when the number of free radicals (also called reactive oxygen species) produced exceeds the ability of your body's antioxidant defence system to neutralise them. This is not a problem at low levels (and can even be beneficial for promoting muscle

adaptations) but, if sustained, it can damage cell membranes and DNA, impair muscle function and hasten fatigue. By consuming a diet rich in antioxidant nutrients (such as vitamins C and E), you will strengthen your body's antioxidant defences and help reduce the damage associated

with oxidative stress. Eating at least five servings per day of a wide variety of fruit and vegetables is the best way to provide your body with the antioxidants it needs. Berries, citrus fruit, dark green leafy vegetables, onions, nuts and olives are all particularly good antioxidant sources.

- **Berries, nuts, red wine** and **dark chocolate** contain polyphenols that encourage the growth of 'good' microbes
- **Try fermented foods containing probiotics –** These are the live bacteria found in non-dairy yogurt, sauerkraut (fermented cabbage), miso (fermented soya bean paste), tempeh (fermented soya beans), kombucha (fermented tea) and kimchi (fermented Chinese cabbage) and will have a short-term beneficial effect on your gut microbiota (it lasts only as long as you are eating these foods regularly)
- **Avoid heavily processed foods –** They contain ingredients, such as emulsifiers, that either suppress 'healthy' microbes or increase 'unhealthy' species
- **Focus on prebiotics –** These are a type of dietary fibre that feed the 'good' microbes in your gut. Consuming more of them will increase the proportion of 'good' microbes. Foods rich in prebiotics include beans, lentils, chickpeas, Jerusalem artichokes, onions, garlic, asparagus and leeks.

Can exercise improve gut health?

There's a growing body of research that suggests many of the benefits of exercise – both physical and psychological – may be attributable to changes in the composition and function of your gut microbiota. It's thought that elite athletes have a unique make-up of gut microbes that are part-responsible for their superhuman performances.

A study led by researchers at the University College Cork in Ireland found that the gut microbiota of elite rugby players was significantly more diverse than that of non-athletes.[35] More recently, researchers were able to identify differences in the composition of the athletes' microbiota sorted by type of sport.[36] This matters because increased microbial diversity is linked to better immunity, higher resistance to upper respiratory tract illness and lower rates of obesity. This can also have a knock-on effect on digestion, weight, mood and chronic disease risk. In another study, scientists at the University of Illinois at Urbana-Champaign found that six weeks of endurance exercise improved the diversity of volunteers' gut microbes.[37] When they stopped exercising, their microbiomes reverted to what they had been at the start of the study. These studies provide compelling evidence

WHAT IS INFLAMMATION?

Inflammation is the body's natural response to protect itself against harm, whether germs, chemicals or toxins. There are two types: acute and chronic. Acute inflammation occurs in response to an injury or illness; your immune system sends out white blood cells to surround and protect the area, creating visible redness and swelling. In these situations, inflammation is essential and beneficial. Chronic inflammation, on the other hand, is not beneficial. It is a longer-lasting immune response that persists over months or years and not only puts you at greater risk of chronic diseases, like heart disease, stroke and type 2 diabetes, but can also increase fatigue during endurance exercise and hamper your recovery afterwards. It is thought that eating too many calories, or too much sugar or fat over time can increase inflammation in the body, while a diet rich in plant foods (particularly polyphenol-rich fruit and vegetables) as well as regular aerobic exercise all help reduce inflammation.

that exercise can induce changes in the gut microbiota independent of diet.

Can a vegan diet help or hinder gut problems?

Gut problems, often called 'runner's tummy' or 'the trots', are common among athletes. It is estimated that 30 to 50 per cent of endurance athletes experience symptoms such as diarrhoea, an overwhelming need to evacuate your bowels, abdominal pain and cramping, belching, bloating, nausea, heartburn, flatulence and vomiting.[38] In a study of recreational runners, 43 per cent reported symptoms in the seven days prior to a marathon and 27 per cent during the race.[39]

We do not know for certain why this happens, but it is likely linked to the reduced blood flow to the digestive organs during high-intensity exercise (known as gastro-intestinal ischemia). During exercise, blood is diverted away from your digestive organs to provide the increased oxygen requirements imposed by your muscles. Unfortunately, this results in the gut slowing down, reduces the gut's ability to absorb nutrients and increases the permeability of the gut, all of which can lead to gut symptoms. In addition, the physical 'jostling' of the intestines during running and increased levels of stress hormones (due to anxiety before a race) affect gut motility and this can further exacerbate the condition. Certain foods and drinks may irritate the gut – for example, high intakes of fibre, fat, protein or fructose.

To overcome gut problems, try keeping a food and symptoms diary to help you identify any trigger foods or drinks. Common culprits include foods that are high in fibre (e.g. beans and lentils), cruciferous vegetables (e.g. cabbage, cauliflower and broccoli) and caffeine, so you may want to avoid them and reduce your fibre intake before an important event. It typically takes one to two days for fibre to pass through the gut, so start cutting down on fibre and switching to white bread, rice and pasta about three or four days before a competition.

However, it is possible to 'train your gut' by consuming carbohydrate foods or drinks during exercise. Start with small amounts, say half a banana, then gradually increase the amount and frequency. This helps increase the number of carbohydrate transporters in your gut so that you become better able to digest and absorb carbohydrate during exercise. Recent research suggests that probiotics may also help alleviate gut problems. A study at Liverpool John Moores University found that runners who took a probiotic supplement for 28 days before a marathon experienced fewer and less severe gut symptoms compared to those who did not take supplements.[40] However, building a healthier gut microbiome may be the best long-term solution (see also 'How can you improve your gut health?' p. 18).

The environment advantage

Avoiding meat and dairy products can also benefit the environment and go a long way towards reducing climate change and cutting your carbon footprint. Vegan diets use significantly less energy, land, pesticides, fertiliser, fuel, feed and water and cause less environmental damage than those with animal products. Livestock are typically fed with plants rich in protein, so if you consume the plant protein directly instead, you avoid the resource inputs required to raise the livestock. For example, to produce 1 kg protein from kidney beans requires 18 times less land, 10 times less water, nine times less fuel, 12 times less fertiliser and 10 times less pesticide compared to producing 1 kg protein from beef.[41] By eating less meat and dairy, you can cut the diet-related environment impact by nearly half.[42]

Animal agriculture is one of the biggest contributors to climate change and responsible for water and air pollution, deforestation, depleted fish stocks, soil degradation, damaged ecosystems and a loss of biodiversity. It accounts for 15–30 per cent of all greenhouse gas emissions that heat up our planet.[43] This is because livestock produce large quantities of methane, nitrous oxide and carbon dioxide. According to a study published in the journal *Science*, producing animal foods, such as meat and dairy, emits 10–50 times more greenhouse gases than most plant foods, such as beans, lentils, fruit and vegetables.[44] They provide just 18 per cent of all calories but take up 83 per cent of farmland and produce 60 per cent of agriculture's greenhouse gas emissions.

In the past decade, a growing body of evidence has emerged, showing that shifting from animal- to plant-based diets lowers emissions of greenhouse gases and thus might be more environmentally sustainable.[45] For example, using calculations based on 210 foods, a study by Swedish researchers estimates that a vegan diet can reduce greenhouse gas emissions and land use by up to 50 per cent.[46]

It is increasingly clear that vegan diets provide a better outcome for both health and the environment. The Eat-Lancet Commission recommends that every country should switch to a more plant-based diet in order to improve global and planetary health.[47] Public Health England's EatWell Guide emphasises plant foods alongside reduced amounts of animal foods. The Carbon Trust estimates that if individuals moved from current eating patterns to the government's EatWell Guide recommendations, a 31 per cent reduction in greenhouse gas emissions, 17 per cent saving on water use and 34 per cent reduction in land use could be achieved.[48]

3

The vegan athlete's plate: how to build a balanced vegan sports diet

Whether you are a keen amateur or elite athlete, the good news is that a well-balanced vegan diet can supply all the energy and nutrients you need to support the physical demands of your sport.

The key is consuming the right amounts and types of different foods that will fuel your workouts and events. To help you do this, I have created the Vegan Athlete's Plate, which can be tailored to the day-to-day fuel demands of your training programme. Produced in line with the UK Vegan Society's Vegan EatWell Guide and the US Olympic Center and University of Colorado Athlete's Plates, it gives you a simple guide to the types and proportions of foods you need to achieve a balanced diet. Each food group supplies a similar profile of nutrients, thus giving you plenty of options and flexibility for planning your meals. It is a good idea to vary your meals as much as possible – the wider the variety of foods you eat, the more likely you are to meet your nutritional needs. The Vegan Athlete's Plate can be adapted to meet the different fuel demands of your training on different days.

Some days may be recovery or easy training days, while others may comprise moderate or hard training. This chapter provides three versions of the Athlete's Plate for different training days.

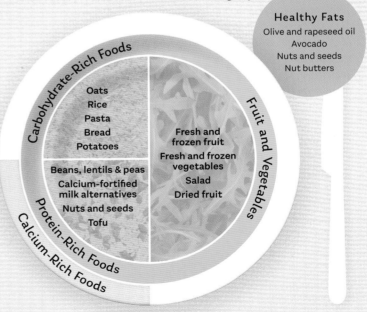

Healthy Fats
Olive and rapeseed oil
Avocado
Nuts and seeds
Nut butters

Carbohydrate-Rich Foods
Oats
Rice
Pasta
Bread
Potatoes

Protein-Rich Foods
Calcium-Rich Foods
Beans, lentils & peas
Calcium-fortified milk alternatives
Nuts and seeds
Tofu

Fruit and Vegetables
Fresh and frozen fruit
Fresh and frozen vegetables
Salad
Dried fruit

THE VEGAN ATHLETE'S PLATE

The Vegan Athlete's Plate divides foods into four main groups:

1 Fruit and Vegetables
2 Protein-Rich Foods
  (including Calcium-Rich Foods)
3 Carbohydrate-Rich Foods
4 Healthy Fats

Fruit and vegetables: Aim to eat at least five portions a day, ideally scaling up to 10 portions of fruit and vegetables if you can. A portion is 80 g of any fresh or frozen fruit or vegetable, or 30 g of dried. For example, one small apple, banana or orange, about six strawberries, three broccoli florets or one carrot. According to a growing body of research, getting beyond the five-a-day minimum and towards 10-a-day could confer added protection against heart disease, certain cancers, as well as performance benefits.[1] Foods in this group are excellent sources of key vitamins and minerals that are vital to life and optimal performance, including vitamin C, beta-carotene, folate and potassium, as well as fibre and phytonutrients. At each meal, aim to achieve a rainbow of colours – green, red, purple, yellow, white and orange – varying them as much as possible. This is because each colour has its unique set of health-promoting phytonutrients, many of which act as antioxidants that help protect cells from damage and reduce inflammation after exercise. As well as varying the colours, try to include different textures, spices and seasonal foods to give your body a wide range of vitamins, minerals and phytonutrients. Buying local and what's in season is environmentally friendly and economical.

Protein-rich foods: Include at least one serving of beans, lentils, chickpeas, soya milk alternative, tofu, tempeh or soya yogurt alternative in each meal. These foods should comprise roughly one quarter of your plate. They are also excellent sources of fibre, iron, zinc and magnesium, while calcium-set tofu and fortified soya milk alternatives also provide calcium. Athletes need more protein than sedentary people so aim for approximately 15–30 g protein per meal (see also p. 32). Mixing different protein sources throughout the day will also mean you get all the amino acids you need.

Calcium-rich foods sub-group: Ensure that you include at least two portions of calcium-rich foods each day: calcium-fortified plant milk and yogurt alternatives and calcium-set tofu (see also p. 27). These count towards your protein-rich foods.

Carbohydrate-rich foods: These include pasta, rice, oats, noodles, potatoes, sweet potatoes, bread and cereals. There is no minimum requirement for carbohydrate so adjust your portion size according to your activity level. The more active you are, the bigger portions you must consume. Whole grains are preferred to refined grains because they contain the entire grain, which means they are richer in fibre, B vitamins and iron.

Healthy fats: These include nuts, seeds, avocado, olive and rapeseed oil. Aim to include one food from this group in most of your meals. Try to include walnuts or seeds rich in omega-3s daily (see also p. 26). Nuts and seeds also provide protein, magnesium, fibre, iron and zinc.

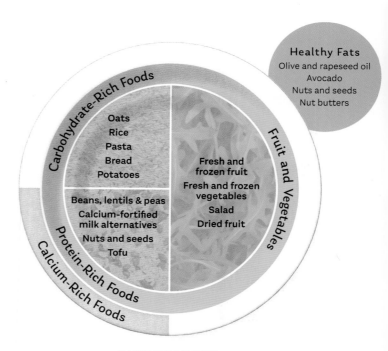

EASY TRAINING

Easy training or recovery days

On easy training days, you may do low-intensity activities such as walking, jogging or yoga. Your fuel and carbohydrate needs will be relatively low. To ensure you get all the nutrients you need, aim for roughly one half of your plate to be made up of fruit and vegetables, roughly one quarter carbohydrate-rich foods and roughly one quarter protein- and calcium-rich foods. Include some healthy fats such as olive or rapeseed oil, nuts, seeds, nut butter or avocado in each meal.

Moderate training days

On moderate training days, you may do moderate- or high-intensity endurance exercise, such as running, cycling, swimming or football, for one to two hours. Your fuel and carbohydrate needs will be higher than on easy training days, so you will need to eat more carbohydrate-rich foods. This will allow you to maintain muscle glycogen stores, sustain your training and prevent early physical and mental fatigue. Divide your plate into thirds and aim to have roughly one third of your meal plate

made up of carbohydrate-rich foods, roughly one third protein- and calcium-rich foods and roughly one third fruit and vegetables. Include some healthy fats, such as olive or rapeseed oil, nuts, seeds, nut butter or avocado, in each meal. You may add extra nutrient-rich snacks (*see also* box on high-energy snacks, p. 25) to meet your increased energy and nutritional needs.

Hard training days

On hard training days, you may do high-intensity endurance exercise, such as running, cycling or swimming, for longer than two hours, or do two moderate- or high-intensity training sessions or events. Your fuel and carbohydrate needs will be very high so you will need to eat more carbohydrate-rich foods. This will allow you to maintain muscle glycogen stores, sustain your training, and prevent early physical and mental fatigue. Aim to have roughly one half of your meal plate made up of carbohydrate-rich foods, roughly one quarter protein- and calcium-rich foods and roughly one quarter fruit and vegetables. Include some healthy fats such as olive or rapeseed oil, nuts, seeds, nut butter or avocado in each meal.

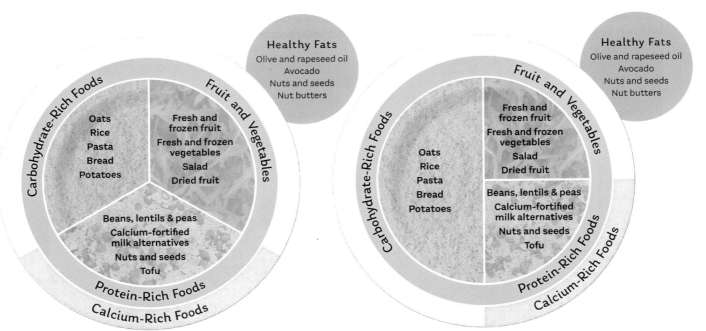

MODERATE TRAINING

HARD TRAINING

persistent fatigue, then ask your doctor for a blood test to check for B12 deficiency.

Omega-3 fatty acids

Omega-3s are vital for heart health and brain function but can also help reduce inflammation and promote recovery after intense exercise. A lack of omega-3s may put you at risk of immune or hormonal dysfunction, which may in turn reduce your performance.

There are three main types of omega-3 fatty acids: eicosapentaenoic acid (EPA), docosahexaenoic acid (DHA) and alpha-linolenic acid (ALA). The main source of EPA and DHA is oily fish, which means vegan diets tend to fall short of omega-3s. However, these long-chain fatty acids can be made in the body from the conversion of ALA into EPA and DHA. Rich sources of ALA include rapeseed oil, ground flaxseed (linseed), hemp, chia and pumpkin seeds (and their oils) and walnuts. One tablespoon chia or ground flaxseed, 2 tablespoons of hemp seeds or six walnut halves daily will supply enough ALA to meet the European Food Safety Authority recommended daily intake of 250 mg. However, since the conversion rate of ALA to EPA and DHA is relatively low, it may be a good idea to take a vegan omega-3 supplement (*see also* p. 30).

Iron

The American College of Sports Medicine states that iron deficiency can impair muscle function and limit exercise performance.[4] Theoretically, vegans may have a higher risk of iron deficiency anaemia since iron from plants is less well-absorbed than that in meat (1–22 per cent vs 15–35 per cent). In practice, this may not happen as the body adjusts absorption according to its iron needs. So, if your iron stores (serum ferritin) are low, the body absorbs a greater percentage of iron from food to replenish them; similarly, when iron stores are 'full' then the body absorbs less.[5] One study found that iron absorption increases ten-fold if you are iron deficient. Furthermore, the body is very efficient in recycling its iron as it renews red blood cells.[6]

Good plant sources of iron include whole grains, quinoa, nuts, seeds, beans, chickpeas, lentils, peas, leafy green vegetables and dried apricots. Table 3.2 gives the iron content of various plant foods. One argument against plant foods as a source of iron is their high content of phytates, which reduce iron absorption. However, these can be removed by soaking (and discarding the water) and cooking, so provided you eat beans, lentils and grains cooked rather than raw, then your body will be able to absorb the iron it needs. Canned beans and lentils are cooked and therefore low in phytates. Furthermore, you can increase iron absorption by pairing any iron-rich food with vitamin C-rich foods, such as red peppers, broccoli, oranges,

TABLE 3.2: THE IRON CONTENT OF VARIOUS PLANT FOODS

Food	Amount of Iron (mg)
5 heaped tbsp (250 g) cooked quinoa (75 g dry weight)	5.9
4 heaped tbsp (200 g) cooked red lentils (75 g dry weight)	4.8
5 heaped tbsp (250 g) cooked wholegrain pasta (75 g dry weight)	3.5
4 heaped tbsp (200 g) canned chickpeas	3.0
100 g tofu	2.7
1 small handful (25 g) pumpkin seeds	2.5
3 tbsp (100 g) spinach	2.1
50 g oats	2.0
2 slices wholemeal bread (80 g)	1.9
4 ready-to-eat dried apricots (50 g)	1.7
3 tbsp (100 g) broccoli	1.7
1 level tbsp (15 g) tahini	1.6
1 small handful (25 g) cashews	1.6

TABLE 3.3: THE CALCIUM CONTENT OF VARIOUS PLANT FOODS

Food	Amount of calcium (mg)
100 g calcium-set tofu	400
200 ml calcium-fortified plant milk alternative	240
150 ml calcium-fortified plant yogurt alternative (plain, Greek-style or sweetened)	180
2 ready-to-eat dried figs (50 g)	115
4 heaped tbsp (200 g) cooked red kidney beans (75 g dry weight)	140
3 tbsp (100 g) kale	130
1 level tablespoon (15 g) tahini	102
4 tbsp (200 g) canned chickpeas	86
1 tbsp chia seeds	72
1 small handful (25 g) almonds	60
2–3 florets (80 g) broccoli	56
3 tbsp (100 g) pak choi (Chinese cabbage)	54

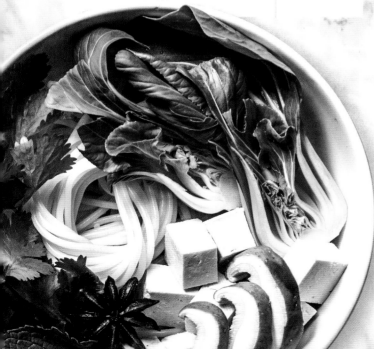

or berries. Vitamin C, or ascorbic acid (along with citric acid also found in fruit and vegetables), enhances iron absorption in the body.

Iron is needed for making haemoglobin, the oxygen-carrying protein in red blood cells. Low levels of iron in your diet can result in iron-deficiency anaemia. Early signs include persistent tiredness, pallor, light-headedness and above-normal breathlessness during exercise. According to the Academy of Nutrition and Dietetics, all athletes, whether vegan or not, are at greater risk of developing iron deficiency compared with non-athletes.[6] That's because aerobic training increases red blood cell manufacture, which in turn increases iron needs. At the same time, iron can be lost from the body via sweat, through gastrointestinal bleeding (which sometimes occurs during very strenuous exercise) and through foot strike haemolysis (destruction of red blood cells caused by repeated pounding of the feet on hard surfaces). Women in general are more susceptible than men to iron deficiency due to iron losses through menstruation.

Calcium

The easiest way to get your calcium quota is by substituting a calcium-fortified plant-based milk alternative for cow's milk. Most brands contain similar amounts to their dairy equivalent – although you will need to check the label. A study published in the *Journal of Nutrition* found that the calcium in plant milk alternatives is absorbed just as well as that in dairy

TABLE 3.4 THE CALCIUM ABSORPTION OF PLANT FOODS

Absorbability	Plant food
Good	Calcium-fortified plant milk and yogurt alternatives, calcium-set tofu, kale, broccoli, pak choi (Chinese cabbage), Brussels sprouts, cauliflower, watercress
Fair	Red beans, white beans, pinto beans
Poor	Sesame seeds, rhubarb, spinach

milk.[7] Other good sources include calcium-set tofu (again, check the label), beans, lentils, peas, green leafy vegetables (spring greens, kale, broccoli and pak choi/ Chinese cabbage), okra, chia seeds, sesame seeds, tahini (sesame seed paste), dried figs and almonds. Table 3.3 shows the calcium content and Table 3.4 shows the absorbability of calcium from various plant foods.

The recommended intake for adults is 700 mg daily. You can get one third of this amount from 200 ml calcium-fortified plant milk or yogurt alternative or about 60 g calcium-set tofu. Spinach is not a good calcium source as it contains oxalate, which reduces calcium absorption.

Calcium is needed for strong, healthy bones and teeth. It also helps with blood clotting and nerve and muscle function. Low intakes over time may result in weak bones and increase your risk of stress fractures and brittle bones (osteoporosis).

Vitamin D

Often called the 'sunshine vitamin', vitamin D is produced in your skin in response to ultraviolet B (UVB) radiation. It is beneficial for bone health, as well as athletic performance and healthy immunity. But one in five people have low levels, which may impair muscle function and strength and increase the risk of injury and illness. A study published in the *British Journal of Sports Medicine* found that more than half (57 per cent) of club athletes were deficient in vitamin D, putting them at greater risk of injury and respiratory infection.[8] Vitamin D supplementation may be beneficial if your blood levels are below 50 nmol/L.

One of the best ways to improve vitamin D levels is to spend time in the sun. Researchers recommend around 10–15 minutes daily sunlight exposure between April and September.[9] This should provide sufficient

TABLE 3.5: THE VITAMIN D CONTENT OF VARIOUS PLANT FOODS

Food	Amount of vitamin D (mcg)
200 ml fortified plant milk alternative	1.50
1 bowl (30 g) fortified bran flakes	1.11–2.52*
1 bowl (30 g) fortified oats	1.29
150 ml calcium-fortified plant yogurt alternative (plain, Greek-style or sweetened)	1.13
100 g UV-exposed mushrooms	5.0

values depend on the brand

year-round vitamin D, while also minimising the risks of sunburn and skin cancer. Vegan sources include fortified foods, such as non-dairy spread, plant milk and yogurt alternatives and certain breakfast cereals, wild mushrooms and mushrooms exposed to UV light (you can do this at home by placing mushrooms in a sunny spot for about half an hour in spring and summer). This is quite a small range

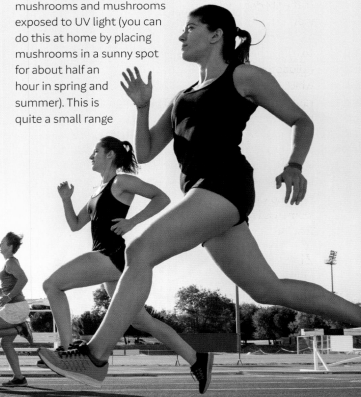

of foods, which makes it difficult to ensure enough vitamin D. For this reason, Public Health England advise taking a daily supplement containing 10 micrograms (mcg) of vitamin D from October to April (*see also* p. 30). Table 3.5 gives the vitamin D content of various plant foods.

Iodine

There are very few plant sources of iodine, so you should either take a supplement (*see also* p. 30) or use a plant milk alternative fortified with iodine, but do check the label as it is not added to all brands. Although seaweed and kelp contain iodine, they are not good options because levels vary and can sometimes be extremely high, which carries a risk of excessive intakes. Excessive iodine can result in thyroid problems. The safe upper limit is approximately 600 micrograms (mcg) per day for adults. Similarly, iodised salt (salt with added iodine), which is available mainly in health food shops, isn't a good option either as you would need to consume large amounts – around 1½ tsp (7.5 g), which is far in excess of the recommended daily upper limit of 1 tsp (5 g) – to get your daily iodine. Most salt sold in the UK does not contain added iodine, though.

Iodine is a mineral that is needed to make thyroid hormones, T3 (triiodothyronine) and T4 (thyroxine), which help regulate the metabolic rate, growth and development. It is especially important during pregnancy for normal brain development in the foetus and for growth in young children. Having low levels can lead to a lower metabolic rate and weight gain, and in pregnant women is linked to lower IQ and reading scores in their children.

Zinc

The best plant sources of zinc include whole grains, beans, lentils, chickpeas, nuts, seeds and quinoa. Table 3.6 gives the zinc content of various foods. As with iron, the phytates found in beans, lentils and the bran layer of whole grains can theoretically reduce the amount of zinc that can be absorbed from food, but provided you consume them cooked then you will be able to absorb sufficient zinc. This mineral is needed for growth and also plays a role in the proper functioning of the immune system, hormone production and fertility. A deficiency may impair your performance. The recommended daily amount is 7 mg for women and 9.5 mg for men.

Which supplements do you need?

Eating a balanced, varied diet that meets your energy needs is the best way of getting your vitamins and minerals. That is because nutrients are better absorbed when consumed as part of whole foods rather than supplements. Having said that, vitamin B12, iron, zinc, calcium, vitamin D and iodine are sometimes in short supply in vegan diets, so if you exclude animal foods completely, you may benefit from specific supplements. Furthermore, athletes have higher nutritional needs

TABLE 3.6: THE ZINC CONTENT OF VARIOUS PLANT FOODS

Food	Amount of zinc (mg)
2 tbsp (30 g) chia seed	1.4
2 tbsp (30 g) pumpkin seeds	2.0
2 tbsp (30 g) cashew nuts	1.8
100 g tofu	1.6
2 tbsp (30 g) ground flaxseeds	1.3
2 slices (80 g) wholemeal bread	1.3
4 heaped tbsp (200 g) cooked lentils (75 g dry weight)	2.0
4 heaped tbsp (200 g) canned red kidney beans	1.4
5 heaped tbsp (250 g) cooked quinoa (75 g dry weight)	2.5
4 tablespoons (200 g) canned chickpeas	1.6
3 tbsp (45 g) oats	1.0

than the general population and may incur higher losses through sweat and tissue damage. You can get a simple blood test to check your nutrient levels from an accredited private provider or your GP. If results show that you have borderline or deficient levels of certain nutrients, then you should seek guidance on supplementation from your doctor or healthcare professional. You may wish to consider the following nutritional supplements. Sports supplements are covered in Chapter 6 (*see* pp. 48–49).

Multivitamins

Multivitamin supplements that provide approximately 100 per cent of the nutrient reference value (NRV) for most nutrients are unlikely to do any harm and may be a convenient insurance against deficient intakes as long as you stick to the dose recommended on the label. This is particularly important for fat soluble vitamins (A, D and E) and all minerals as excessive levels can accumulate in the body and cause toxicity. Risk of toxicity is lower for water-soluble vitamins (B and C) as any excess is excreted in your urine. You should also check that the nutrient levels in other supplements you take do not overlap with those in your multivitamin supplement. However, there is no evidence that consuming more vitamins and minerals than you need results in better health or performance.

Vitamin B12

You will need to get your vitamin B12 either from fortified foods or supplements. You can, of course, combine more than one option as there is no harm in exceeding the nutrient reference value (NRV). The Vegan Society recommends either a daily supplement providing at least 10 micrograms (mcg) of vitamin B12, or a weekly B12 supplement providing at least 2000 micrograms (mcg).[10] This provides a similar absorbed amount to consuming 1 microgram (mcg) three times a day from fortified foods. The less frequently you obtain B12, the more B12 you need to take as B12 is best absorbed in small amounts. There are two types of vitamin B12, but cyanocobalamin is recommended as it is the most stable type.

Vitamin D

Public Health England recommends taking a supplement of 10 micrograms (mcg) or 400 IU vitamin D from October to April to maintain good immunity and safeguard against deficiency.[11] If you are unsure whether you are getting enough vitamin D, you can have your blood levels tested by your GP or an accredited private provider. Deficiency is usually judged as having a serum level below 30 nmol/l and insufficiency between 30 and 50 nmol/L, meaning supplements may be beneficial.[12] There are two forms of vitamin D: D2, derived from yeast, is typically used in fortified foods, while D3 is more effective in raising blood levels than D2 so this is the best option. Ensure your D3 supplement is labelled as suitable for vegans. Some D3 supplements are made from lanolin in sheep's wool but fortunately, vegan supplements made from algae are widely available.

Omega-3s

Although your body can convert alpha-linolenic acid (ALA) into eicosapentaenoic acid (EPA) and docosahexaenoic acid (DHA) (*see also* p. 26), it may not produce enough, so it is worth considering a vegan omega-3 supplement. Look for fish-free supplements made from algae oil, which will provide a natural and concentrated form of both EPA and DHA. This is particularly important if you are pregnant or breastfeeding as omega-3s are needed for the baby's brain development.

Iron

If you have been diagnosed with iron deficiency, then you will benefit from iron supplements. Symptoms include persistent tiredness, fatigue, above-normal breathlessness during exercise and loss of endurance and power. Your doctor can carry out a simple blood test (that measures ferritin, haemoglobin, iron and haematocrit) and will prescribe supplements if you need them. However, if you are not deficient, then you should not take supplements above the Recommended Dietary Allowance (RDA) as high doses cause side effects such as constipation.

Iodine

The most reliable way to meet your iodine needs is a multivitamin supplement containing the recommended daily requirement for iodine, 150 micrograms (mcg).

4

Protein: all you need to know

'Where do you get your protein?' is probably the most common question every vegan gets asked. Although protein deficiency is extremely rare in Western countries, many athletes worry that a vegan diet cannot supply enough protein or think that they need to take protein supplements every day. Fortunately, the research says otherwise and there is an easier way to think about how (and where) you get your protein on a vegan diet.

What is protein needed for?

This essential macronutrient helps build and repair cells, including muscles, cartilage and ligaments. It also makes skin, bones, hair and lots of other tissues, as well as enzymes, hormones and antibodies for your immune system. Although most of the energy used during exercise comes from carbohydrate and fat, protein also contributes to the fuel mixture, to the tune of 2–5 per cent, although this can be as high as 15 per cent in situations where you're low on carbohydrate – for example, in the latter stages of a long, high-intensity endurance workout or event.[1]

How much protein do athletes need each day?

There is no doubt that athletes need more protein than the average person, with the American College of Sports Medicine, Academy of Nutrition and Dietitians of Canada recommending an intake of between 1.2 and 2.0 g/kg body weight/day.[2] For a 70-kg athlete, this

equates to between 84 to 140 g per day – approximately double the daily protein recommendation for the general population (0.75 g/kg body weight/day or 53 g for a 70-kg person). Following endurance exercise, this extra protein is needed to build mitochondrial proteins, the powerhouses of the muscle cells that make energy.

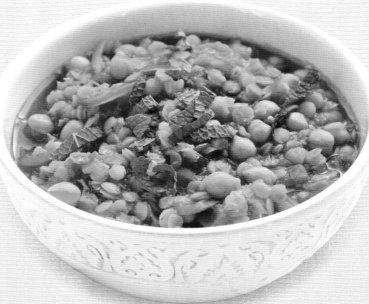

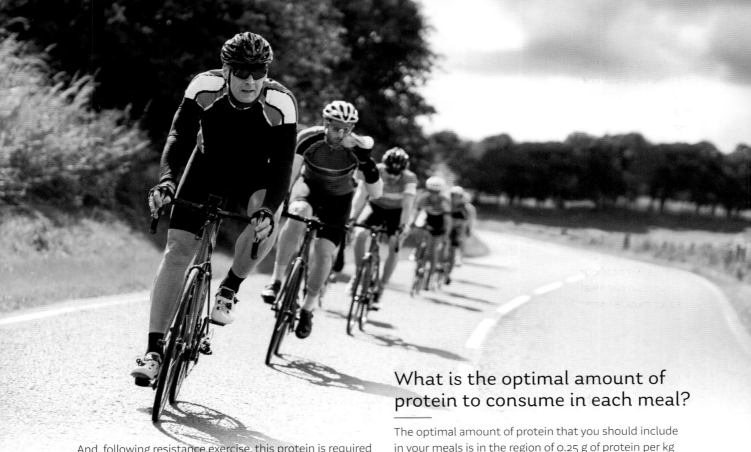

And, following resistance exercise, this protein is required for building muscle mass.

In practice, the exact amount you need will depend on the type, intensity and duration of your activity, as well as your body composition goals. So, if you do mostly endurance activities, then your protein requirement will be closer to the lower end of the range (1.2–1.4 g/kg body weight). But for building muscle mass, and for optimal performance and recovery following strength and power activities, an intake within the upper end of the range (1.4–2.0/kg body weight) would be more appropriate.[3] If you are aiming to lose body fat, then you will need additional protein – between 1.2 and 1.6 g/kg body mass – to prevent or offset some of the muscle mass loss that occurs during a calorie deficit.[4] Protein also promotes satiety and has been shown to improve appetite control and weight management. If you know where to get your protein from and use the Vegan Athlete's Plate in Chapter 3 (see p. 21), then there is no reason why you cannot meet your protein needs.

What is the optimal amount of protein to consume in each meal?

The optimal amount of protein that you should include in your meals is in the region of 0.25 g of protein per kg of body weight, or an absolute amount of 20 g protein.[3,5] You may need slightly more, around 40 g, in your post-workout meal if you have done a whole-body resistance workout.[6] Over-60s may also benefit from slightly higher protein intakes – in the region of 0.4 g protein/kg of body weight/meal – to help counteract the anabolic resistance that occurs as we get older.[7] In practice, think of 20 g as a ballpark figure, though, and adjust this depending on your body weight, activity and age. In Part 2: Recipes, all the main meal recipes supply at least 20 g protein either on their own or with the suggested accompaniment.

Is protein timing important?

The timing and distribution of your protein intake throughout the day is also important. Studies have shown that consuming protein *soon after exercise* and then *evenly spacing* protein across your meals promotes better muscle recovery, mass and strength gains than consuming it unevenly across meals.[8] That's because the 'anabolic window' after exercise isn't confined to just a few hours, as once thought, but extends at least 24 hours, so muscle repair and manufacture take place continuously.[9] Aim to consume similar amounts of protein at breakfast, lunch and dinner. This may require quite a big change in your eating habits if, like most people, you tend to get most of your protein at dinner or eat relatively little at breakfast.

Is too much protein harmful?

Consuming more protein than you need is not harmful, but nor is it beneficial. Protein uptake and utilisation plateaus out at about 0.4 g/kg body weight or around 40 g protein per meal – exceeding this does not produce greater muscle mass, strength or performance gains. Any surplus protein is simply broken down and used for energy or excreted in your urine.[10]

How can vegan athletes get enough protein?

The answer is that most plant foods contain *some* protein, which means you can easily obtain all the protein your body needs from many sources. These include:

Legumes: beans, lentils, peas, chickpeas, peanuts
Soya products: soya milk alternative, soya yogurt alternative, edamame beans, tofu, tempeh (fermented soya beans), soya mince
Grains: bread, pasta, rice, oats, bulgur (cracked) wheat, teff, freekeh, spelt, seitan (wheat protein)
Pseudo-grains:* quinoa, amaranth, buckwheat
Mycoprotein: Vegan Quorn
Nuts: walnuts, cashews, almonds, pecans, Brazils, pistachios and nut butters
Seeds: sunflower, sesame, pumpkin, flax, hemp and chia seeds

Pseudo-grains are not true grains – they are seeds from plants that are not classed as cereal grasses. However, they have a similar nutrient profile and are cooked and eaten in a similar way to other grains

That is quite a long list of foods! You may be surprised to learn that many foods that are often regarded as carbohydrate-rich, such as pasta, bread and oats, are also valuable sources of protein. For example, an average portion of pasta (75 g) provides 9 g of protein, the same as an average portion (125 g) of beans or lentils. Even vegetables contain some protein: an average-sized potato (175 g) contains 3 g and an average portion of broccoli (80 g) contains 4 g. So, if you eat a portion of pasta, beans and broccoli, then you will be getting 22 g protein – the amount deemed optimal for muscle building.[5] Additionally, you will be getting plenty of vitamins, minerals, fibre and phytonutrients, which promote health, performance and recovery. Table 4.1 (p. 35) gives the protein content of various plant foods within different food groups. With so many options available, it is clear that you do not need to consume animal protein to meet your requirements.

You may find it more challenging at first to eat enough protein on a vegan diet compared with a diet based on animal foods, since most plant foods contain less protein per 100 g of food. This is because they also contain other nutrients such as carbohydrate and unsaturated fat, as well as fibre, which 'dilute' the protein. This means that you will need to eat larger amounts of plant foods to get the same amount of protein as you would in animal foods. Eating bulkier meals may feel difficult at first, but rest assured, your body soon adapts. A great tip is to include tofu (12–18 g/100 g) and tempeh (21 g/100 g) in several of your meals each week as they are more concentrated protein sources. Try Pad Thai with Crispy Tofu (*see* p. 122), Tofu Satay Skewers (*see* p. 151) or Teriyaki Tempeh Noodle Bowl (*see* p. 105).

When it comes to substituting dairy milk, soya is the best option out of all plant-milk alternatives (*see* p. 60), containing around seven times more protein than other varieties. And if you are buying soya yogurt alternative, go for a concentrated type – Greek-style contains nearly 6 g of protein per 100 g, roughly double that of the original version.

What is the difference between animal and plant proteins?

Plant and animal proteins differ in their content of amino acids, as well as their digestibility. Both of these factors dictate how useful the protein will be to the body and how much of it will be converted into body proteins. This is sometimes called 'protein quality' and replaces the outdated notion of complete and incomplete proteins. It is a popular misconception that plant foods are lacking in certain amino acids (*see* p. 11 – myth 3) – all plant foods contain all 20 amino acids, including the nine essential amino acids.[11, 12, 13]

Our bodies need all nine EAAs in the right ratios similar to the way a house needs all of the right building materials in the right proportions to be built. Generally speaking, animal protein sources (e.g. dairy and meat) provide EAAs in ratios closely matched to the body's requirements.[14] Hence they are considered to be high-quality. In contrast, there is only a handful of high-quality plant sources of protein, i.e. that contain all nine EAAs in relatively high amounts, namely soya (e.g. soya milk alternative, soya yogurt alternative, tofu, tempeh and

miso), quinoa, buckwheat, amaranth, chia and hemp seeds. But that does not mean that you should only eat these foods in order to fulfil your protein needs. Eating a wide variety of other plant foods throughout the day will also ensure you get all nine EAAs. Beans, lentils, peas, grains and nuts contain smaller amounts of one or more EAA – sometimes called the limiting amino acid – but you can easily compensate by consuming more than one plant food in the same 24-hour period.[11, 15] For example, beans are relatively low in methionine, while grains are relatively low in lysine (*see box* 'How to Get Enough Lysine', p. 35) and nuts are low in threonine. Eating beans, rice and nuts will give you all nine EAAs.

Protein quality is not always the bottom line, though. Many plant protein sources come with a package of other nutrients, such as carbohydrate, fibre, vitamins, minerals and phytonutrients. Many of these components are not found in animal protein sources, which is why many health authorities, including the World Health Organization (WHO) and Food and Agriculture Organization of the United Nations (FAO), Public Health England's (PHE) Eatwell Guide, the EAT-Lancet Commission and the British Dietetic Association recommend prioritising plant foods in their dietary recommendations.

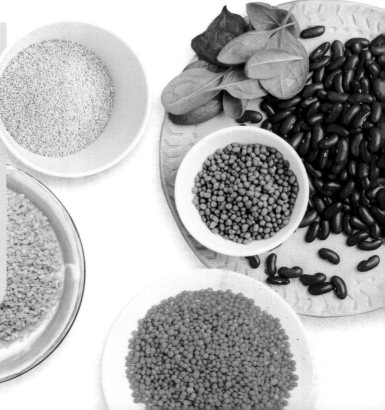

AMINO ACIDS

When we talk about protein, we are really talking about amino acids, the building blocks that make up proteins. In total, there are 20 types of amino acids that can be combined in many different ways to make hundreds of different proteins, each with specific roles in the body. Amino acids are classified either *essential or non-essential*. There are nine *essential amino acids (EAAs)* that the body cannot make and therefore must be provided by the diet. Non-essential amino acids, on the other hand, can be created in the body, so they are not essential for us to consume. It is the amounts of these EAAs in foods relative to the body's requirements that determine how useful the protein is to the body.

Are plant proteins less digestible than animal proteins?

Plant proteins are slightly harder to digest than animal proteins. This is because the fibre and other plant components make it harder for digestive enzymes to break down proteins. However, soaking beans and lentils, or cooking grains make plant proteins easier to digest and improves their overall protein quality. The digestibility of proteins can be measured by a score called the Digestible Indispensable Amino Acid Score (DIAAS),[16] which measures how many amino acids are digested in the small intestine. Generally, animal proteins have DIAAS values greater than 100, while plant proteins have DIAAS values less than 75, with the exception of soya protein, which is between 75 and 100 and oats around 75. Table 4.1 shows the DIAAS values of various animal and plant foods.[14]

HOW TO GET ENOUGH LYSINE

Lysine is considered a 'limiting amino acid' in vegan diets as it is not found in high quantities in most plant foods. If you do not get enough, the absorption and utilisation of other amino acids is reduced. One of the building blocks of carnitine, essential for converting fat into energy, it helps the body make collagen and plays an important role in supporting the immune system. The richest vegan sources are soya products (milk and yogurt alternatives, tempeh and tofu); beans, lentils, peas, chickpeas; buckwheat, quinoa, wild rice; cashews, pistachios; pumpkin, flax, chia and hemp seeds; and vegan Quorn and seitan.

TABLE 4.1: THE PROTEIN QUALITY (DIAAS) OF VARIOUS FOODS[14]

Food	Protein Quality (DIAAS)
Animal protein sources	
Milk	114
Egg	113
Plant protein sources	
Soya protein isolate	98
Black beans	59
Green lentils	65
Chickpeas	83
Peanuts	43
White rice	57
White bread	29

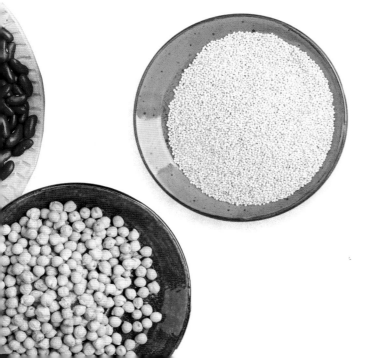

Are plant proteins as good as animal proteins for building muscle?

Previously, plant proteins were considered less effective than animal proteins for muscle building due to their lower protein quality. However, this is no longer the case. According to the Academy of Nutrition and Dietetics, vegetarian and vegan diets provide the same protein quality as meat-based diets.[18] A review of studies published in the *International Journal of Sport Nutrition and Exercise Metabolism* in 2018 found that plant proteins are equally effective as animal proteins, provided you eat them in sufficient amounts.[19] The researchers concluded that soya and whey protein supplements produce similar gains in strength and muscle mass following resistance training.

There was no difference in 1 rep-max bench press nor squat strength or total lean body mass gains between those consuming whey and those consuming soya supplements.

Furthermore, a meta-analysis published in the *British Journal of Sports Medicine* of studies in 2017 found that once you get to 1.6 g/kg body weight/day, the source of your protein, animal or plant, makes no difference.[20] More recently, a study at the University of São Paulo and McMaster University compared gains in leg muscle mass and strength between vegans and omnivores consuming 1.6g protein/ day for 12 weeks.[21] Researchers found no difference in gains between the groups, suggesting that plant proteins are just as effective as animal proteins for building muscle providing they are consumed in sufficient quantity.

These findings appear to go against the findings of previous studies, which suggested soya was less effective than animal proteins for building muscle, at least on a gram-for-gram basis.[22] However, this is due to its lower content of leucine, an essential amino acid thought to be an important trigger and substrate for muscle building.[23] But if you were to consume more soya protein so that you matched the leucine content of whey, then the differences would likely disappear. In other words, provided you consume enough leucine (i.e. reach the 'leucine threshold'), then it does not matter whether this comes from animal or plant sources.

How can you increase the muscle-building properties of plant proteins?

You can increase the muscle-building potential of plant protein with the following strategies:

1 Eating larger quantities of protein. Researchers suggest that consuming slightly more protein per meal will increase the conversion into muscle protein and thus enhance the potential of plants to support muscle growth and strength.[17, 24] All the main meals recipes in this book supply a minimum of 20 g protein.

2 Eat foods rich in leucine, such as tofu, beans, lentils, nuts and seeds. This will increase the overall protein quality of your meal and increase its muscle-building potential. For example, you can get 2 g leucine, an amount thought to be optimal for muscle building, from either 140 g tofu or 30 g soya protein isolate (*see* Table 4.2, p. 38, which shows the amount of leucine in various foods).

3 Eating a variety of plant proteins over the course of a day. This will provide a more balanced amino acid profile and means that the shortfall of EAA in one source will be compensated by higher amounts found in another. Although you do not have to combine proteins in the

HOW TO GET ENOUGH LEUCINE

Leucine is one of the nine essential amino acids that are needed by the body. It is particularly important for those wanting to build strength and muscle mass because it triggers the process of muscle building.[25] Once inside a muscle cell, leucine stimulates the so-called mTORC1 (mammalian target of rapamycin)

signalling pathway, which results in the formation of new muscle proteins. To maximise muscle building, a 'leucine threshold' must be surpassed, which the International Society of Sports Nutrition estimates to be between 0.7 and 3 g of leucine or about 20–40 g of protein.[3] The richest vegan sources of leucine are soya-

based protein powders, tofu and tempeh (*see* Table 4.2, p.38). Beans, lentils, chickpeas, oats, nuts and seeds also provide good amounts. However, plant proteins generally have a lower concentration than animal proteins, so you will need to consume relatively high amounts to get the optimal amount of leucine for muscle growth.

same meals, many food combinations happen naturally in meals, including the following examples:

- Three-Bean Chilli with Cashew Cream (p. 134)
- Puy Lentil Salad with Harissa-Roasted Cauliflower and Walnuts (p. 98)
- Courgette, Edamame and Asparagus Pasta (p. 124)
- Red Lentil Dal with basmati rice (p. 127)
- Lentil Tabbouleh (p. 87)
- Mixed Grain Salad with Crispy Tempeh and Harissa Dressing (p. 92)
- Porridge made with soya milk alternative
- A falafel wrap
- Peanut butter on toast

Should you take protein supplements?

Whole foods are generally a better option than supplements. Not only do they supply a range of other nutrients, the interaction of the other nutrients contained within the food matrix may actually increase the use of protein for muscle repair. The International Association of Athletics Federations recommends whole-food sources of protein rather than supplements, although this does not take into account the needs of vegan athletes.[26] In practice, vegan diets can be very bulky, making it difficult for some athletes to get enough protein. In these cases, protein supplements may be a helpful addition. They may also be a convenient option if you are training or competing in an environment where your usual foods are not available or there is no opportunity to store or prepare foods.

There is a wide variety of plant protein supplements available, including soy, pea, rice and hemp protein powders. Soy protein is a good option as it contains a balanced amino acid profile and relatively high levels of leucine compared with other plant proteins. Alternatively, opt for blends of plant proteins, such as pea and rice protein, as they contain a

THE FUTURE OF PLANT PROTEINS

Scientists are trialling a number of other strategies to increase the anabolic potential of plant proteins. These include the fortification of plant protein sources with EAAs, such as leucine, lysine and methionine, which are typically present in relatively low amounts; making plant protein blends; and selectively breeding plants (genetic manipulation) to improve their amino acid composition. If these strategies prove successful, then they may offer a commercially viable way of reducing the global demand for animal protein and moving to a more sustainable food supply.

more balanced amino acid profile than single plant proteins. Protein powders can be added to shakes, porridge or yogurt, or mixed into cookie dough, pancake or cake batter to boost your protein intake. While supplements can help meet your daily requirement, there is no evidence that consuming more protein than you need will lead to greater muscle mass, strength or performance gains.

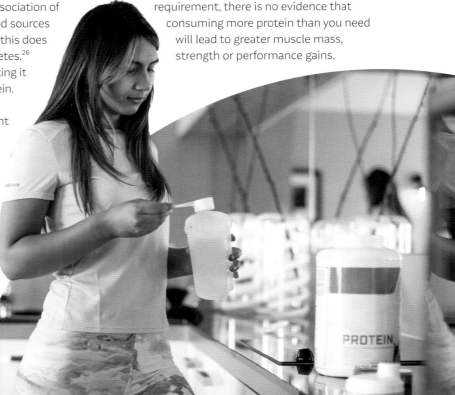

TABLE 4.2: THE PROTEIN AND LEUCINE CONTENT OF VARIOUS FOODS

	Food	Portion	Amount of protein (g)*	Amount of leucine (g)**
Protein Supplements	Soya protein isolate powder	1 scoop (25 g)	23	1.7
	Vegan protein blend powder	1 scoop (25 g)	18	n/a
	Pea protein powder	1 scoop (25 g)	20	n/a
Soya products	Soya milk alternative	200 ml	7	0.4
	Greek-style soya yogurt alternative (plain)	200 ml	12	n/a
	Soya yogurt alternative	200 g	8	n/a
	Firm tofu	100 g	13	1.4
	Marinated tofu pieces	100 g	18	n/a
	Tempeh	100 g	21	0.6
	Soya mince (frozen)	100 g	15	n/a
Pulses	Red kidney beans (canned)	125 g drained weight (half a 400 g can)	9	0.6
	Chickpeas (canned)	125 g drained weight (half a 400 g can)	9	0.8
	Edamame beans (frozen)	125 g	15	0.9
	Puy lentils (cooked)	125 g	14	0.8
	Green or brown lentils	125 g drained weight (half a 400 g can)	8	0.8
	Red lentils (cooked)	125 g	9	0.8
	Peas	125 g	7	0.4
	Hummus	2 tbsp (50 g)	3	0.2
	Falafel	4 falafel (88 g)	8	0.8
Nuts	Peanuts	2 tbsp (30 g)	9	0.5
	Peanut butter	2 tbsp (30 g)	9	0.5
	Walnuts	2 tbsp (30 g)	5	0.4
	Cashews	2 tbsp (30 g)	6	0.4
	Almonds	2 tbsp (30 g)	6	0.4
	Pecans	2 tbsp (30 g)	3	0.2

	Food	Portion	Amount of protein (g)*	Amount of leucine (g)**
Nuts cont.	Almond butter	2 tbsp (30 g)	8	0.4
	Almond milk alternative	200 ml	1	0
Seeds	Sunflower seeds	2 tbsp (30 g)	7	0.5
	Pumpkin seeds	2 tbsp (30 g)	9	0.7
	Flaxseeds	2 tbsp (30 g)	6	0.4
	Chia seeds	2 tbsp (30 g)	6	0.4
	Sesame seeds	2 tbsp (30 g)	7	0.4
	Tahini	2 tbsp (30 g)	7	0.4
Grains	Oats	75 g uncooked	9	1.0
	Oat milk alternative	200 ml	1	
	Pasta	75 g uncooked (150 g cooked)	9	0.3
	Wholewheat noodles	75 g dry uncooked (200 g cooked)	9	n/a
	Rice noodles	75 g dry, uncooked (200 g cooked)	7	0.3
	Basmati rice	75 g dry, uncooked (200 g cooked)	6	0.4
	Wholemeal bread	2 slices (80 g)	8	0.5
	Rye bread	2 slices (80 g)	7	0.5
	Bulgur (cracked) wheat	75 g uncooked (200 g cooked)	9	0.6
	Seitan (wheat protein)	100 g	18	n/a
Pseudo grains	Quinoa	75 g dry, uncooked (200 g cooked)	10	0.6
	Buckwheat	75 g dry, uncooked (200 g cooked)	6	0.6
Myco protein	Quorn vegan fillets	1 fillet (63 g)	9	n/a
	Quorn vegan pieces	70 g	11	n/a
Vege-tables	Potatoes	1 medium (175 g)	3	0.2
	Broccoli	3 florets (80 g)	4	0.1

*Data from UK Composition of Foods Integrated Data Set and UK manufacturers' data
**Data from the US Food Database
n/a = data not available

5

Peak performance: what to eat and drink before, during and after exercise

What, how much and when you eat makes a big difference to your performance and recovery. Maintaining proper hydration is also crucial if you want to get the most out of your training.

This chapter builds on the Vegan Athlete's Plate described in Chapter 3 (*see* p. 21), providing you with an easy guide to pre-, mid- and post-workout fuelling. It will help you tailor your food intake to your workout or event training, whatever time of day you exercise.

Pre-workout fuelling

A pre-workout meal will raise blood glucose and provide energy for your workout. This will help delay the onset of fatigue and increase your endurance and performance, as well as keeping hunger at bay. However, you will also need to consider your carbohydrate intake in the previous 24–48 hours as most of the energy expended during your workout will come from your stores of carbohydrate (glycogen) and fat.

What should you eat before?

The best foods to eat before exercise depend on your workout goals and individual preference, but the boxes on p. 41 give you some suitable pre-workout meal and snack options. Your pre-workout meal should be easy to digest and include foods rich in carbohydrate (e.g. rice, oats, pasta or potatoes), with smaller amounts of protein-rich foods and healthy fat. This combination of macronutrients will provide sustained energy to help get you through your workout. Both protein and fat slow the digestion and absorption of carbohydrate, so the closer your meal is to

PRE-WORKOUT MEALS

- A pitta bread filled with falafel and avocado
- A baked potato with hummus and roasted vegetables
- Maple, Pecan and Cranberry Granola (p. 76) with plant milk alternative
- Black Bean and Sweet Potato Salad (p. 88)
- Rainbow Stir-Fry (p. 125)
- Spiced Chickpea Pilaff with Almonds and Coconut Yogurt (p. 130)
- Beans and Greens Salad with Pesto (p. 84)
- Moroccan-Spiced Chickpea Soup (p. 94) with toasted pitta bread
- Sweet Potato, Beetroot and Chickpea Salad (p. 104)
- Satay Noodles (p. 128)

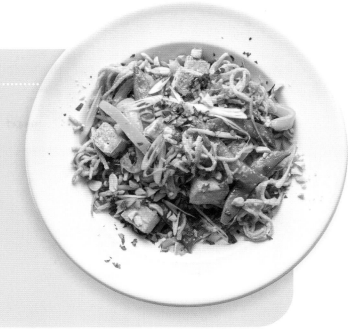

your workout, the less protein or fat you should eat. On the other hand, eating a meal devoid of fat and protein could leave you hungry and lacking in energy. It is usually a good idea to avoid large amounts of fibre-rich foods within 30 minutes of exercise, especially if you are prone to gut issues or feel nervous before an event. Fibre slows stomach emptying, which can make you feel full and uncomfortable. However, moderate amounts of fibre eaten two to four hours or longer before exercise should not pose a problem and according to a handful of studies may even be advantageous for endurance as fibre prevents spikes in blood glucose and insulin during exercise.[1]

Pre-workout snacks

- Bananas or any other fresh or dried fruit
- Toast with peanut butter and banana
- Fruit and nut bars
- Oat cakes or crackers with hummus
- Cinnamon Apple Granola Bars (p. 70)
- Jumbo Oat Cookies (p. 190)
- Power-Up Cinnamon Coffee Smoothie (p. 202)
- Seeded Banana Muffins (p. 196)

long an interval to cause this energy to be used up by the time you begin exercising. Eating a meal too close to exercise may result in stomach discomfort and indigestion as the blood supply is shunted away from your gut to your muscles. On the other hand, leaving too long a gap means you may feel hungry, light-headed and lacking energy during exercise. You should feel comfortable – not too full and not hungry.

The closer your pre-workout meal is to your workout, the smaller it must be. If you have less than two hours before your workout, opt for an easy-to-digest snack. Anything more substantial may result in gut issues and discomfort during exercise. In practice, the exact timing of your pre-workout meal will probably depend on practical constraints such as work hours and travel. Try to plan meals as best you can around these commitments. For example, if you work out at 6 o'clock in the evening, either schedule lunch around 2 p.m. (leaving you a four-hour

How long before exercise should you eat?

Ideally, try to schedule your pre-exercise meal so that you have a two- to four-hour gap before your workout. This will give you enough time to digest the food but not too interval before your workout) or around midday and then eat a snack between 4 and 5.30 p.m. (leaving you a 30-minute to two-hour interval).

How much should you drink before exercise?

It is important to ensure that you are properly hydrated before you begin exercising. This will help you perform at your best and reduce the risk of dehydration and exercise-related illness during your workout. You can get a good idea of your hydration status by checking the colour of your urine: it should be pale straw-coloured, not deep yellow, and should not have a strong odour. A darker colour indicates that you may be dehydrated and, therefore, need to drink more.

The American College of Sports Medicine advises drinking 5–10 ml/kg body weight, equivalent to 350–700 ml for a 70-kg athlete, in the two to four hours before exercise.[2] Sip little and often during the hours beforehand rather than gulping a large volume just before you start. This will allow your body to use the fluid most effectively and avoid the need to go to the toilet or have any stomach discomfort during your workout.

Water is the best option before most workouts but if you also need a source of fuel (e.g. where a pre-workout meal or snack is not available or feasible), then sports drinks would be a good option as they provide carbohydrate as well as fluid.

Mid-workout fuelling

If you are exercising for less than 60 minutes, then you do not need to consume extra fuel. Stay on top of your hydration needs, though, and drink water when you need to. For endurance exercise longer than 60–90 minutes, you may benefit from consuming carbohydrate during your workout or event. This will help maintain your blood glucose levels and supply a quick source of energy to your muscles. Precious glycogen stores will be conserved, which means you will be able to continue exercising for longer before reaching fatigue.

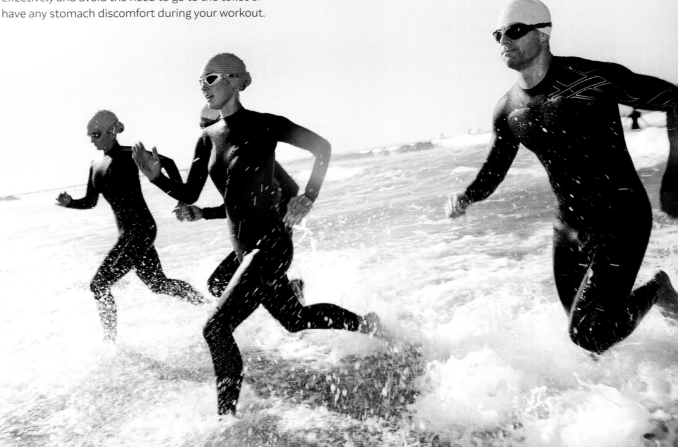

When should you fuel?

Start fuelling approximately 45–60 minutes into your workout or event, depending on your exercise intensity and hunger. If you are exercising at a high intensity or feel hungry then you may need to consume carbohydrate earlier. It takes 15–30 minutes for the carbohydrate you have consumed to reach your muscles, so do not wait until you are exhausted before you begin fuelling. The key is to consume carbohydrate little and often; avoid over-eating, but don't avoid eating altogether. Most athletes prefer to consume fuel approximately every 30 minutes, although you may find a slightly different interval will suit you better.

What should you consume?

Aim to consume between 30 g and 60 g carbohydrate per hour (or 15–30 g every 30 minutes), depending on your exercise intensity and duration.[2,3] If you are exercising at a low intensity, then you probably won't need more than 30 g/hour. If you are exercising at a high intensity, then you can experiment with higher amounts, closer to 60 g/hour, and see how your body responds. This may be in the form of whole foods (e.g. bananas, dried fruit, fruit and nut bars, or homemade bars and balls) or sports foods (e.g. sports drinks, energy bars, gels or chews, p. 48), depending on your personal preference. Some options for foods and drinks providing 30 g carbohydrate are given above. The maximum amount of glucose the body can absorb is 60 g/hour, so don't overconsume carbohydrate as it won't aid your performance. Instead, it will 'sit heavy' on your stomach and may trigger unwanted gut symptoms, such as nausea, bloating and diarrhoea.

There is an exception, though, when you are exercising at a high intensity for longer than two and a half hours – for example, during long, hard endurance events. In these situations, consuming up to 90 g carbohydrate

> ### Foods and drinks providing 30 g carbohydrate
>
> - One large banana (150 g)
> - 500 ml isotonic sports drink (6 g carbohydrate/ 100 ml)
> - Two (40 g) Medjool dates
> - A small handful (40 g) of raisins
> - 2 x 35 g fruit and nut bars*
> - One or two (45 g) cereal bars*
> - One (45 g) energy bar*
> - Four (40 g) energy chews*
> - One (50 g) energy gel*
> - Four Brownie Energy Balls (p. 174)
> - Four Almond and Chocolate Chip Energy Bites (p. 170)
>
> *Depending on the brand

per hour from a mixture of glucose (or maltodextrin) and fructose can improve your endurance. Studies have found that drinks or foods containing a mixture of glucose (or maltodextrin) and fructose in a 2:1 ratio allows the body to absorb carbohydrate faster and therefore supply the muscles with more carbohydrate than glucose-only drinks.[4,5] This is clearly an advantage during events such as marathon and ultra-running, endurance cycling and triathlons, when your energy needs are high and prolonged. Energy drinks, gels and bars providing a 2:1 mixture of glucose and fructose are widely available, but many wholefoods, including fresh and dried fruit also supply a similar ratio.

For long workouts or races, you may prefer to take savoury as well as sweet options to reduce flavour fatigue and the risk of tooth damage. Good options include bite-sized sandwiches, wraps, rolls or pitta filled with yeast extract or nut butter, rice cakes or crackers. Consuming fat-rich foods such as nuts is unlikely to help performance during most workouts as fat cannot be turned into energy fast enough but may help reduce hunger and slow stomach emptying during ultra-distance events.

What should you drink?

For workouts lasting less than an hour, water is usually the best option. If you are exercising longer than an hour, consuming extra carbohydrate in the form of a sports drink (p. 48) or diluted fruit squash, cordial or juice will not only hydrate your body but also help maintain blood glucose levels. Alternatively, you may prefer consuming water plus food (e.g. bananas, raisins or gels). And if your sweat losses are high and prolonged – for example, during endurance activities longer than two hours, or

HYPONATRAEMIA

Hyponatraemia is rare but can occur during endurance events, such as marathons and ultra-distance races. It happens when the concentration of sodium in your blood falls to an abnormally low level (<130mmol/L) and can be caused by drinking too much water or by losing excessive sodium in your sweat. When this happens, your body's water content increases and your cells begin to swell. Early warning signs include headache, nausea, bloating, water retention, disorientation and confusion. In extreme cases, it can result in seizures, coma or death. To prevent such problems, ensure you do not drink more fluid than you lose through sweating and only to the point at which you are maintaining, not gaining, weight. If you are sweating profusely for long periods (e.g. >1.2 l/h for longer than two hours) and/or produce very salty sweat, then you will need to consume additional sodium, either in the form of an electrolyte drink or salty foods (such as pretzels) with water.

when exercising in hot and humid conditions – you may also benefit from sodium (electrolyte) replacement in the form of sports drinks or electrolyte tablets (p. 48). Sodium helps the body absorb and retain fluid more effectively than water. Excessive losses of sodium during exercise can result in hyponatraemia, a potentially dangerous condition (*see box*, above).

How much should you drink?

There are no hard and fast rules about how much you should be drinking during exercise. Your sweat rate (and therefore your fluid needs) is highly variable and will depend on the intensity and duration of your exercise, your fitness, altitude and the surrounding temperature and humidity. For example, you will lose more fluid during intense and prolonged exercise, and in hot and humid conditions.

Dehydration – generally defined as a body water deficit of 2–3 per cent of your weight – will increase your core body temperature and cause increased stress on your heart and lungs. When this happens, exercise will feel harder, stamina, speed and performance will drop and fatigue develops, all of which can amount to a reduction in endurance and performance.[6] You may also experience headaches, nausea and dizziness.

Ideally, you should replace most of your fluid losses so that you limit your body fluid deficit to less than 2 per cent of your body weight. This is equivalent to a weight loss of 1.4 kg for a 70-kg athlete. Anything greater than this will negatively impact your health and performance. For workouts where sweat losses are relatively small, simply drinking to thirst will prevent dehydration as well as hyponatraemia. However, where potential sweat losses are high – for example, during prolonged endurance activities in hot and humid climates – you will need to be more proactive in your drinking strategy to avoid becoming dehydrated. Scientists recommend an intake of 500–1000 ml per hour for marathon runners, depending on your pace (the faster you run, the more fluid you will need), but you should adjust this amount according to your individual needs and intolerance.[7,8] Drink at regular intervals, but do not force yourself to drink or drink excessively. Trial different hydration strategies in training so that you will know what works best when it comes to competition.

Post-workout refuelling

Good nutrition in the post-workout period will help your muscles recover, restore glycogen more quickly and rebuild themselves stronger. There are three goals of nutrition recovery, also known as the '3 Rs of recovery':

1 Rehydrate
2 Refuel
3 Repair

1 **Rehydrate with fluid and electrolytes.**
The exact amount you need to drink depends on how much fluid you have lost during exercise. You can calculate your fluid loss by weighing yourself before and after training. For optimal rehydration, aim to replace each 1 kg of weight (sweat) loss with 1.25–1.5 l fluid.[2] If your fluid losses have been relatively small, then water will do a perfectly good job at replacing lost fluid. But if fluid losses have been high, then opt for a drink containing sodium, such as a sports or electrolyte drink. Alternatively, water with salty food (e.g. toast with yeast extract) will work equally well and promote more effective fluid retention than water alone. Replacing lost fluid after exercise takes time and is best achieved by drinking little and often. Drinking a large volume in one go stimulates urine formation, so much of the fluid is lost rather than retained.

2 **Refuel with carbohydrate.** Depleted glycogen (carbohydrate) stores need to be replaced after exercise. Failure to do so will result in cumulative fatigue and under-performance in your next workout. The exact amount you need to consume will depend on the type, intensity and duration of your activity, but as a rule of thumb, you will need to consume more carbohydrate after a high-intensity or prolonged endurance workout than after a short- or low-intensity workout. If you train twice a day or have less than eight hours between workouts, then take advantage of the two-hour post-exercise recovery window when glucose will be converted into glycogen 1½ times faster than normal. Aim to consume 1.0–1.2 g of carbohydrate per kg body weight (60–72 g for a 60-kg athlete) each hour for four hours after exercise to maximise glycogen storage.[2] This way, you will ensure your glycogen stores are restored as fully as possible before your next workout. If this amount of

Recovery meals

- A wrap filled with falafel and hummus
- Blueberry and Lemon Protein Overnight Oats (p. 65)
- Cannellini Bean, Cauliflower and Squash Traybake (p. 114)
- Teriyaki Tempeh Noodle Bowl (p. 105)
- Black Pepper Tofu with Pak Choi and Cashews (p. 112)
- Thai Green Curry with Crispy Tofu Balls (p. 133)
- Tofu Satay Skewers (p. 151)
- Tomato and Coconut Dal with Crispy Tofu and Cashews (p. 136)
- Lentil Tabbouleh (p. 87)
- Pad Thai with Crispy Tofu (p. 122)
- Three-Bean Chilli with Cashew Cream (p. 134)

carbohydrate is too much for you, then include some protein too as this will enhance glycogen storage. If you have longer than eight hours between workouts, then then there is no urgency to consume carbohydrate straight after training.[9] You should be able to restore glycogen by including carbohydrate in your normal meals. Provided you consume enough carbohydrate over a 24-hour period, your muscles will recover before your next workout.

3 **Repair with protein.** Consuming protein after a workout helps to repair damaged muscle cells and build new muscle. Your post-workout meal or snack should include 0.25 g protein per kilogram of body weight, depending on your body weight, age and the type and intensity of exercise you have done (*see* p. 32).[10] But tailor this to suit your workout and your body weight. You'll need more following a strength or

Recovery snacks

- Toast with nut butter
- Soya milk alternative and a banana
- A handful of mixed nuts and dried fruit
- Fluffy Banana Protein Pancakes (p. 72)
- Fruit and Granola Yogurt Pot (p. 74)
- Berry Smoothie Bowl (p. 64)
- Mixed Berry Chia Smoothie (p. 203)
- Strawberry Cashew Smoothie (p. 202)
- Tofu Scramble (p. 80)
- Toast with Chickpea Hummus (p. 188)
- Chocolate Protein Bars (p. 184)
- Protein Balls (p. 194)
- Peanut Butter Bars (p. 192)
- Cinnamon Apple Granola Bars (p. 70)

LOW-CARBOHYDRATE HIGH-FAT DIETS

There is long-standing controversy about whether low-carbohydrate, high-fat (LCHF) diets enhance endurance performance. Since we have far more energy stored as fat than glycogen, the thinking is that restricting carbohydrate intake will force the muscles to burn more fat. In theory, this may allow you to fuel long-distance events mostly with fat, reducing the need to consume carbohydrate during the event. Indeed, studies show that these practices may enhance your fat-burning ability and increase the number of mitochondria (the powerhouses that burn fat) in your muscle cells.[12] However, there is no evidence that this results in

improved endurance performance. On the contrary, studies have consistently shown that it makes exercise feel harder at any given intensity and reduces the body's ability to use carbohydrate for fuel during high-intensity exercise, which means you lose some of your ability to produce bursts of energy – for example, in a sprint finish.[13] In a series of studies, dubbed the Supernova studies, Australian researchers have shown that a LCHF diet reduces your energy efficiency (which means you require more oxygen to exercise at any given intensity) and impairs high-intensity endurance performance.[14,15] It also increases cortisol (stress hormone), which

lowers immunity, making you more susceptible to infections.

A more effective strategy for elite athletes is 'carbohydrate periodisation', whereby you perform your low-intensity workouts with low-carbohydrate availability (i.e. consume no carbohydrate before or during exercise) and your high-intensity workouts with high carbohydrate availability (i.e. consume carbohydrate before or during exercise).[16] However, this strategy is not relevant for non-elite athletes as they will gain greatest benefit from a well-planned, balanced diet following the principles in this chapter and Chapter 3 (*see* pp. 21–30).

whole-body workout than following an endurance workout, but generally, a meal containing around 20 g protein is considered optimal for muscle recovery.[11] Ideally, in the immediate post-workout period, you want 'high quality' protein that contains all nine essential amino acids in ratios closely matched to the body's needs – and one that's rich in the amino acid leucine (see p. 36).

Suitable plant foods include soya products (e.g. soya milk alternative, soya yogurt alternative, tofu and tempeh), quinoa, chia and hemp seeds. Beans and lentils are also rich in leucine. Eating a variety of plant proteins over the course of the day will also help your muscles recover faster before your next workout (see p. 36). See the boxes on pp. 45 and 46 for suitable recovery meal and snack options.

FASTED TRAINING

Fasted training means training in a fasted state, i.e. after not eating for 10–14 hours, and is typically done in the morning before breakfast when your glycogen stores are slightly depleted. Similar to training on a low-carbohydrate high-fat diet (*see box* p. 46), the idea behind it is that you will burn a higher percentage of energy from fat. Theoretically, this may promote weight loss or endurance training adaptations. This is true up to a point, but it does not necessarily mean you will lose weight. To lose weight, you need to be in a calorie deficit. In other words, you must consume fewer calories than your body needs over the course of several days, not in a single workout. Fasted training does not necessarily make you burn fat instead of carbohydrate; your body may turn to protein instead and result in a loss of muscle. Studies show that people can exercise longer when they consume a pre-exercise meal than when they fasted.[17] Additionally, fasting makes exercise feel harder so may compromise exercise intensity and volume, resulting in a lower overall calorie expenditure.[18] On the other hand, if you prefer training fasted (e.g. first thing in the morning), then that's fine provided you're doing low- or moderate-intensity exercise (as you'll be burning relatively more fat and less carbohydrate). However, if you plan to do high-intensity exercise for longer than an hour, then having a high-carbohydrate snack 30–60 minutes beforehand will help increase your endurance (as you will be burning relatively more carbohydrate and less fat).

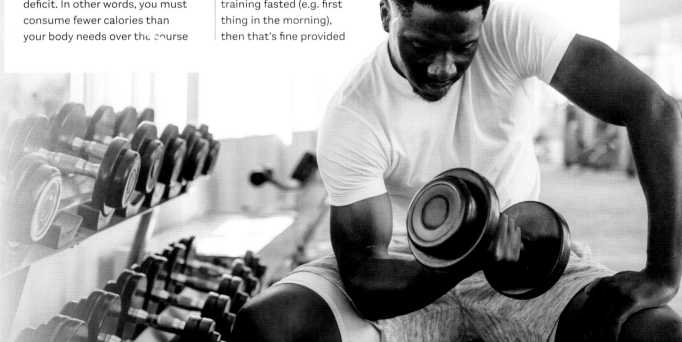

Sports foods and supplements

There is a bewildering array of sports foods and supplements available. Here is a guide to the products that provide either convenient fuelling options or a performance advantage.

Sports foods

Sports foods are a category of dietary supplements that provide energy or nutrients in a more convenient form than whole foods and are designed to be consumed around exercise. While you should aim to meet the majority of your nutritional needs from whole foods, there are certain situations where sports foods may be more practical – for example, if you're training or competing in an environment where there's no opportunity to store or prepare foods, or when your training schedule makes it difficult to do so.

Protein drinks and bars

Protein supplements will not necessarily give you bigger muscles but can be a useful option if you find it difficult to meet your daily protein needs from food alone or simply as a convenient and portable post-workout option to whole food (*see also* p. 37).

Sports drinks

As well as hydration, the sugars in these drinks provide fuel, which can help maintain blood sugar levels during endurance exercise (*see* p. 43). They typically contain 5–8 g sugars/100 ml and electrolytes such as sodium, so may be beneficial during high-intensity endurance exercise lasting longer than 60–90 minutes or immediately after exercise to promote rehydration and refuelling (*see also* p. 45).

Energy drinks

Energy drinks provide sugars and caffeine (*see also* p. 49) and may enhance performance during high-intensity endurance exercise lasting longer than 60–90 minutes.

Energy bars

Energy bars comprise mainly carbohydrate (sugar and maltodextrin) and can provide a fast and convenient mid-workout fuelling option for endurance workouts longer than 60–90 minutes. Whole-food alternatives include bananas, raisins and dates.

Energy gels and chews

Like energy bars, gels are a convenient on-the-go fuelling option for exercise longer than 60–90 minutes and are designed to provide energy quickly, but make sure you drink enough water with them to reduce the risk of stomach upset. Isotonic gels made from maltodextrin are generally better tolerated and digested faster than thick, concentrated gels.

Electrolytes

Electrolyte replacement in the form of drinks or tablets could be useful when sweat losses are high and prolonged – for example, during high-intensity endurance exercise for longer than two hours, or when you are exercising in hot and humid conditions. They promote rapid water uptake by the body and aid fluid retention, so may help avoid hyponatraemia (p. 44) as well as promote rapid rehydration after exercise.

Sports supplements

Sports supplements are a category of dietary supplement designed to enhance performance and are taken in higher doses than you would normally be able to get from food or drink. According to a recent consensus statement by the International Olympic Committee, only very few of these are supported by robust research and offer marginal performance gains.[1] These include caffeine, creatine, beetroot juice and beta-alanine. If you decide to use them, always check that they comply with anti-doping guidance (*see* below) and trial them during training, not on competition day.

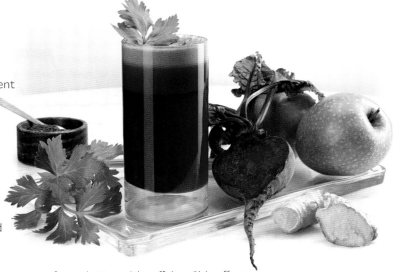

Caffeine

Caffeine may reduce perceptions of fatigue, increase alertness and allow exercise to be sustained at an optimal intensity for longer, potentially enhancing your performance in endurance, anaerobic and strength activities, and those involving repeated sprints. Individual responses vary and not everyone performs better with caffeine. Side effects include tremor, anxiety, sleeplessness, increased heart rate and raised blood pressure.

Creatine

Creatine supplements may improve performance in repeated high-intensity exercise with short recovery periods and, thus, may help increase strength, power and muscle mass. You may experience greater benefits from creatine supplements than non-vegans because you will not be getting any from your diet – creatine is found only in meat and fish. There are several forms of creatine, but creatine monohydrate is the most effective and well-researched form.

Beetroot juice

Beetroot juice, a rich source of nitrate, can improve performance in endurance exercise lasting 12–40 minutes, as well as in repeated high-intensity exercise. It increases the production of nitric oxide in the body, which helps to dilate blood vessels, improve blood flow and reduce the oxygen cost of exercise.

Beta-alanine

Beta-alanine increases the muscles' buffering capacity and, thus, may improve performance during high-intensity anaerobic exercise that would otherwise be limited by a build-up of acidity (hydrogen ions), i.e. events ranging from 30 seconds to 10 minutes, or those involving repeated high-intensity sprints.

ANTI-DOPING GUIDANCE

Dietary supplements are the biggest cause of inadvertent doping in the UK. Unlike prescription medicines, there is no systematic regulation of supplements, which means there is no official check on safety, quality or whether they are free from prohibited substances. The World Anti-Doping Agency (WADA) have a policy of strict liability, which means that each athlete is strictly liable for any banned substance found in their body, taken intentionally or not. You can cut this risk by making sure that your supplement comes from a reputable company with strict manufacturing controls and has a certificate to prove it has been batch tested for banned contaminants by a recognised sports anti-doping lab. Look for the Informed Sport logo on the label and cross-reference the batch number on their website.

PART

2
Recipes

8

Before you begin cooking

Whether you already enjoy a vegan diet, or you simply want to try some new vegan dishes, then the recipes in this section will help you put vegan sports nutrition into practice. They have been created to deliver maximum levels of nutrients as well as delicious fresh flavour.

I have ensured that every dish is packed with the vital nutrients you need to train, recover and perform. Each main meal recipe provides at least 20 g protein per serving, which is the optimal amount needed for muscle growth and recovery (*see also* p. 32).

For each recipe, I have highlighted the key nutritional, health and performance benefits and provided a nutritional breakdown for energy, protein, fat, saturated fat, carbohydrate, total sugars and fibre. This information is intended to help you gain a greater understanding of what you are eating and provides reassurance that each meal is nutritionally balanced. It is not necessary to count calories or track your 'macros', however.

All the recipes are quick and easy to prepare, requiring minimal skill and relatively little effort. Everything you need is widely available from supermarkets so you will not have to go searching for specialist ingredients. You will see that there is plenty of flexibility within each recipe and you do not need to stick rigidly to the ingredient lists. I have given suggestions for alternatives wherever possible so you can use different ingredients according to what you have available or what you fancy.

I believe that fresh ingredients and minimally processed foods should form the backbone of a healthy vegan sports diet. They are naturally filled with vitamins, minerals, fibre and phytonutrients, so will benefit your health, performance and recovery. I have not included meat substitutes ('fake' meats, p. 58) in my recipes as they are heavily processed and often very high in salt. I have also avoided coconut or palm oil and products made with them (e.g. vegan cheese) as they are extremely high in saturated fat (*see also* p. 56).

As far as serving sizes go, the number suggested in each recipe should be regarded as a guide. Everyone has different energy and nutritional needs, so you may need to adjust the amount you need according to your appetite. I am a great believer in saving time wherever possible, so I have devised a

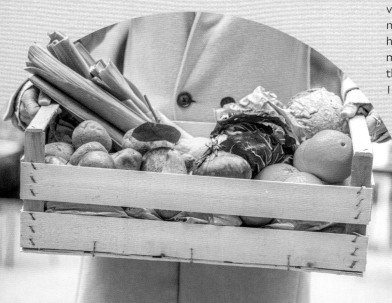

whole chapter of one-pot dishes (Chapter 11, pp. 106–137) that can be prepared ahead and eaten later. These can all be batch-cooked – halve or double up the quantities if you wish – and stored in containers in the fridge (usually for up to three days) or freezer (usually for up to three months).

Metric measurements are given in the recipes but you'll find conversion charts for imperial and cup measurements at the end of the book.

Vegan ingredients

Stocking up with a few healthy and versatile ingredients is a great first step to vegan cooking. Here is a guide to some popular vegan foods, many of which are included in the recipes in this book. Try adding one or two new ones to your shopping basket each week and build up your vegan larder gradually.

Agave syrup

Agave syrup is extracted from the sap of the agave plant, a type of cactus native to Mexico. It has a slightly thinner consistency than honey and can be used on porridge or as an alternative to sugar, honey or maple syrup in baking. It contains less glucose and more fructose than sugar, so has a lower glycaemic index (GI) – meaning it is absorbed more slowly into the bloodstream. However, it contains the same amount of energy (calories) as sugar and should be consumed only in moderation.

Aquafaba

Aquafaba is the liquid that you usually drain off from canned chickpeas (or other beans). It has a protein structure similar to that of egg whites, which means it can be whipped into semi-stiff peaks. It can be used to make meringues, Yorkshire pudding and macaroons or added un-whipped to cookies and mayonnaise. To make meringues, simply whisk with 1 teaspoon cream of tartar or a drop of lemon juice using an electric whisk for five minutes. Then add an equal amount of sugar, spoon by spoon, whisking between each addition of sugar.

Almond milk alternative

Almond milk alternative is made from ground almonds and water. However, most brands contain relatively very small amounts of nuts – around 2 g per 100 ml, the rest being mainly water. This means that almond milk alternative is low in protein compared to cow's milk (less than 1 g/100 ml vs 3 g/100 ml), so you will need to get your daily protein from other sources, such as tofu, beans and lentils. Slightly sweet, nutty and creamy, it is good for drinking straight from the carton or used in porridge, desserts and smoothies but is a little too sweet for savoury dishes. It is easy to make your own almond milk alternative: soak 150 g almonds in water overnight, drain and rinse, then process with 900 ml water in a high-speed blender. Strain through a cheesecloth or muslin nut bag, then add vanilla extract or sugar to taste if you wish.

Beans, lentils and peas (pulses)

All pulses are rich in protein, iron, magnesium and B vitamins, as well being an excellent source of fibre, which feeds the healthy microbes in your gut (see p. 17). The recommended daily fibre intake is 30 g, but the average person consumes only 18 g.[1] Eating beans regularly will promote a healthy and diverse gut microbiome, which can affect your exercise performance through improved immunity, faster recovery and lowered inflammation. A healthy gut microbiome also improves the body's ability to gain energy and nutrients from the food we eat.

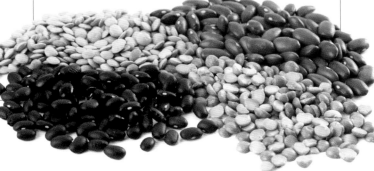

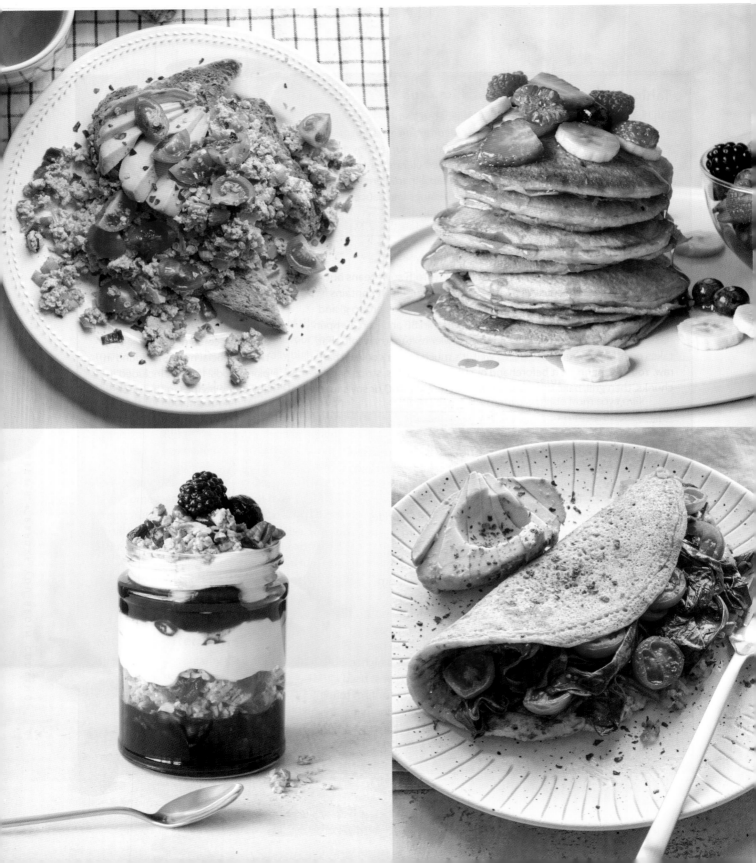

Breakfasts and brunches

Clockwise from top left: Tofu scramble; Fluffy banana protein
pancakes; Chickpea omelette; Fruit and granola yogurt pot.

Berry smoothie bowl

. . . .

Smoothie bowls make a super-speedy breakfast and are a delicious way of getting at least two of your five-a-day. As the name suggests, they are essentially a smoothie served in a bowl and topped with nutrient-rich ingredients, such as nuts, seeds, fruit or granola. This recipe combines four different plant protein sources: chia seeds, almond butter, vegan protein powder and coconut yogurt, ensuring a full complement of essential amino acids to promote muscle growth. It is also rich in vitamin C, fibre and omega-3 fats. Feel free to vary the toppings depending on what you have to hand.

SERVES 1

1 small banana, peeled, sliced
    and frozen
100 g frozen berries (e.g.
    raspberries, blackberries or
    blueberries)
½ scoop (15 g) chocolate vegan
    protein powder (optional)
1 tbsp chia seeds
1 tbsp almond butter
125 ml coconut yogurt
    alternative
125 ml coconut milk alternative

TOPPINGS

Fresh berries, a handful of
granola, walnuts, flaked almonds,
pecans, coconut flakes or mixed
seeds

Add all the ingredients except the toppings to a blender and process until smooth. Pour into a cereal or dessert bowl and top with any combination of berries, granola, nuts, coconut flakes or seeds.

NUTRITION per serving | **420** cals | **25** g protein | **18** g fat (**4** g saturates) | **35** g carbs (**19** g total sugars) | **12** g fibre

Blueberry and lemon protein overnight oats

·············

Overnight oats are the perfect breakfast solution for busy mornings because they can be prepared ahead of time and will keep you fuelled until lunchtime. Simply mix the ingredients the night before, pop in the fridge and overnight they will magically transform into a delicious, creamy and nutritious porridge! The big protein boost comes from protein powder and Greek-style soya yogurt alternative, which contains twice as much protein as other soya yogurt alternatives. I like adding blueberries as they are rich in anthocyanins, which promote muscle recovery, but feel free to swap for any of the alternative toppings suggested below.

SERVES 1

50 g rolled oats
120 ml oat milk
2 heaped tbsp plain Greek-style
   soya yogurt alternative
½ scoop (15 g) vegan vanilla
   protein powder (optional)
2 tsp chia seeds
Zest of ½ lemon
2 tsp maple syrup
75–100 g blueberries (fresh
   or frozen)

OPTIONAL TOPPINGS

Extra blueberries, nuts,
seeds or nut butter

Simply mix all the ingredients together in a bowl, mason jar or jam jar. Cover with cling film or, if you are using a jar, close the top and pop in the fridge overnight.

In the morning, stir, add a splash more milk if you wish (the oats soak up quite a lot of liquid), then top with extra blueberries or any of the suggested toppings.

VARIATIONS

- *Banana and raisin:* Replace the blueberries and lemon zest with a sliced banana, a handful of raisins and a pinch of ground cinnamon.

- *Tahini:* Omit the blueberries and lemon zest. Stir 1–2 tablespoons tahini and 2 chopped Medjool dates into the oats. Serve with fresh fruit.

- *Apple cinnamon:* Omit the blueberries and lemon zest. Cook one roughly chopped apple with ½ teaspoon cinnamon and 2 tablespoons water for 3–5 minutes. Transfer to a separate bowl and leave in the fridge overnight. Top the oats with the apple mixture.

- *Peanut butter:* Stir 1 tablespoon peanut butter (or any other nut butter) into the oats, leave overnight and then top with 1 tablespoon chopped nuts or seeds.

NUTRITION per serving | **478** cals | **26** g protein | **12** g fat (**2** g saturates) | **60** g carbs (**19** g total sugars) | **12** g fibre

Blueberry and banana protein baked oats

· · · · · · · · · · · · · ·

No time to cook porridge every morning? Here is the perfect solution: baked oats.
It's easy to make ahead and a batch will last you all week. Packed with protein and full of
fibre, it will keep you feeling full and satisfied all morning. Soaking the oats helps to soften
them, reduces the baking time and allows the oats to absorb more flavour. The recipe
can be varied countless ways by adding grated apple, walnuts, chocolate chips or raisins
(*see* Variations below). The bars will keep for up to three days in the fridge. Alternatively,
freeze in individual portions and just reheat in the microwave.

SERVES 4

180 g rolled oats
500 ml boiling water
2 bananas
1 tbsp chia seeds mixed with
    1 tbsp water
2 tbsp maple syrup
1 scoop (25 g) vanilla vegan
    protein powder (optional)
100 g fresh or frozen blueberries,
    plus extra for the topping
    (optional)
40 g flaked almonds
2 tsp cinnamon
1 tsp baking powder
250 ml plant milk alternative
    (any type)

Preheat the oven to 180°C/fan 160°C/gas mark 4. Meanwhile, line
a 20 cm square tin with baking paper.

Put the oats and boiling water into a mixing bowl. Allow to stand for
10–15 minutes.

Meanwhile, peel and mash 1½ bananas in a separate bowl until as
smooth as possible. Slice the remaining ½ banana for the topping.
Stir in the chia seed mixture, maple syrup and protein powder (if using).
Pour this mixture over the softened oats and stir to combine.

Add the remaining ingredients to the bowl and stir well. Pour the oat
mixture into the prepared tin and smooth the top. Top with the banana
slices and extra blueberries if you wish. Bake for 35–40 minutes until
golden brown. Allow to cool slightly (it will firm up as it cools), then cut
into squares.

VARIATIONS

· ·

- ***Apple and walnut:*** Add a peeled and diced apple instead of the
blueberries and a handful of walnuts instead of the almonds.

- ***Chocolate:*** Substitute 1 scoop chocolate protein powder or cacao
powder for the vanilla protein powder and add 50 g chocolate chips or
cacao nibs.

- ***Raisin:*** Add 50 g raisins instead of blueberries to the mixture.

NUTRITION
per serving | **383** cals | **16** g protein | **12** g fat (**1** g saturates) | **50** g carbs (**17** g total sugars) | **7** g fibre

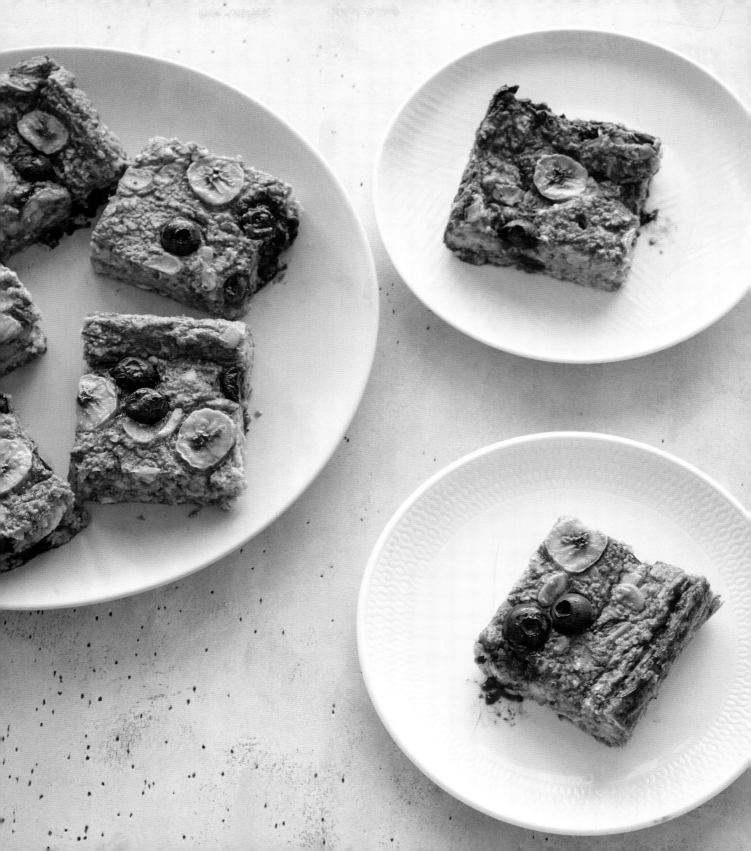

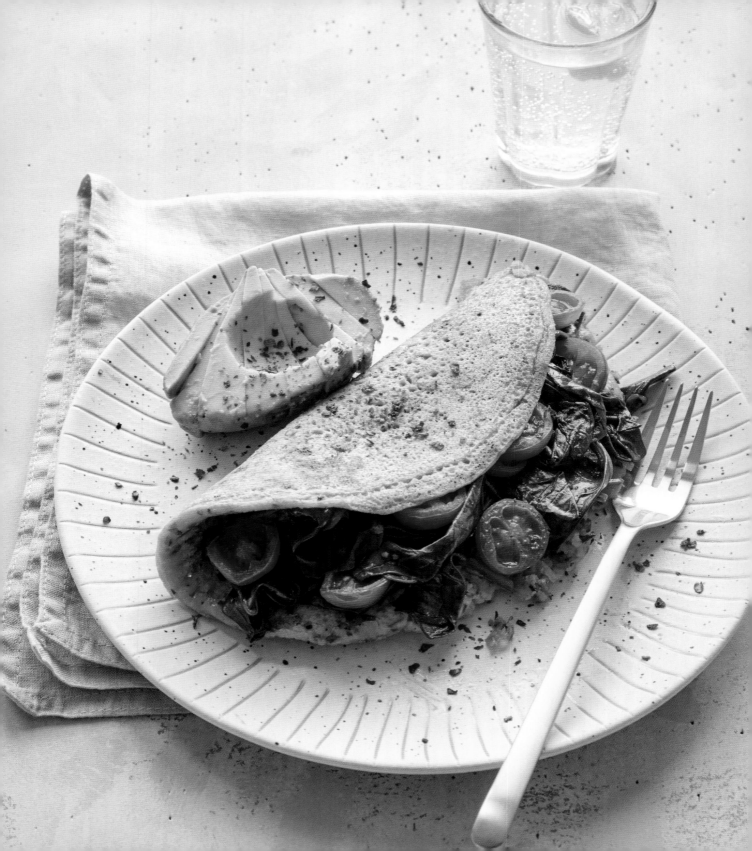

Chickpea omelette

....

If you thought that egg-based dishes like omelettes were off the menu on a vegan diet, then think again! With a few adjustments, it is perfectly possible to recreate your favourite breakfast dish. This omelette is made with chickpea (gram) flour, which is widely available from supermarkets. It's a brilliant egg substitute for vegans as it is rich in protein, fibre and iron. I have filled the omelette with tomatoes and spinach, but you could add chopped red onions, mushrooms, red peppers or peas.

SERVES 1

60 g chickpea (gram) flour
¼ tsp salt
⅛ tsp baking powder
A pinch of turmeric, paprika
  and nutritional yeast flakes
125 ml plant milk alternative
  (any type)
A small handful of chopped
  fresh herbs (e.g. parsley,
  chives or basil) or 1 tsp dried
  mixed herbs

FOR THE FILLING

2 tsp olive oil
6 cherry tomatoes, halved
A handful of baby spinach

TO SERVE

½ small avocado, peeled,
  pitted and sliced
Pinch of chilli flakes

Whisk together in a bowl the chickpea (gram) flour, salt, baking powder, turmeric, paprika and yeast flakes, and milk alternative until smooth. Add the herbs, stir to combine, then leave to stand for a few minutes.

Meanwhile, make the filling: heat 1 teaspoon of the olive oil in a non-stick frying pan over a medium heat, add the tomatoes and cook for a few minutes. Add the spinach, then remove from the heat and set aside.

Wipe out the frying pan and heat the remaining 1 teaspoon oil over a medium heat. When hot, pour in the batter and tip the pan so it spreads out thinly over the base. Cook gently until the top sets and bubbles appear on the surface. Spoon the filling onto one half of the omelette, then fold the other half over using a spatula. Press down with the spatula to seal it and allow to cook for another minute.

Slide the omelette onto a plate and serve with avocado slices and a sprinkle of chilli flakes.

| NUTRITION per serving | **463** cals | **20** g protein | **22** g fat (**4** g saturates) | **40** g carbs (**8** g total sugars) | **11** g fibre |

Cinnamon apple granola bars

· · · · · · · · · · · · ·

These granola bars make a perfect pack-and-go breakfast when you want to head out early for a workout. Packed with oats, nuts and seeds, and sweetened naturally with apples and dates, they guarantee long-lasting energy as well as tasty way of boosting your intake of fibre, omega-3s, iron and zinc. I like to make a batch, then wrap individually in foil so I always have a supply of healthy breakfast bars. They can be stored in the fridge for up to a week in an airtight tin.

MAKES 16 BARS

2 eating apples, peeled, cored and roughly chopped (any variety)
125 g Medjool or soft dates, pitted
100 g nut butter (any type)
100 ml plant milk alternative (any type)
45 g ground flaxseeds
175 g rolled oats
2 tsp cinnamon
75 g pumpkin or sunflower seeds
75 g walnuts, chopped (optional)

Preheat the oven to 180°C/fan 160°C/gas mark 4. Meanwhile, line a 20 cm square baking tin with baking paper.

Add the apples, dates, nut butter and milk to the bowl of a food processor and process until you have a smooth purée. Transfer to a large bowl, add the remaining ingredients and mix together to combine.

Press the mixture into the prepared tin and bake for approximately 30 minutes until the mixture is firm and golden brown. Allow to cool for 10 minutes and then cut into 16 bars.

NUTRITION per bar | **191** cals | **6** g protein | **11** g fat (**1** g saturates) | **15** g carbs (**7** g total sugars) | **3** g fibre

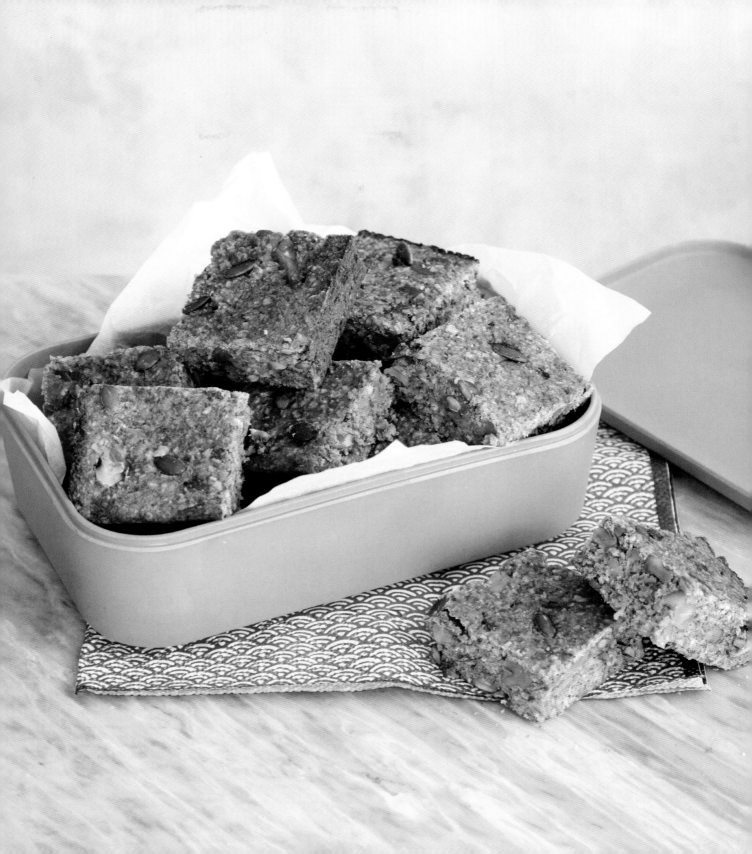

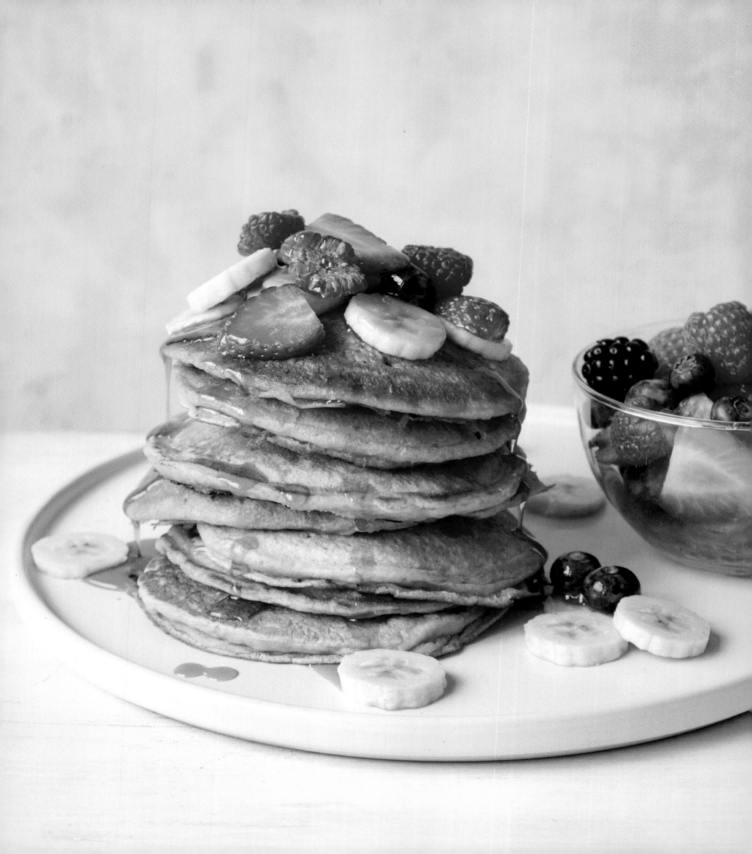

Fluffy banana protein pancakes

· · · · · · · · · · · · ·

These fluffy pancakes are a delicious way to get your protein at breakfast – without using eggs. Instead, I have used vegan protein powder and baking powder, which make the pancakes nice and fluffy. You'll get 20 g protein from four pancakes. Wholemeal flour is a healthier option than white flour as it is higher in fibre, protein and iron.

MAKES 8

250 ml plant milk alternative (any type)
1 scoop (25 g) vegan protein powder (any flavour)
1 ripe banana, peeled and mashed (optional)
1–2 tbsp maple syrup or sugar
2 tbsp light olive or rapeseed oil, plus extra for frying (or use cooking spray oil)
125 g plain or wholemeal flour
1 tbsp baking powder

TO SERVE

Fresh berries (e.g. blueberries, strawberries, raspberries, or blackberries), banana slices, nut butter or maple syrup

Place all of the pancake ingredients in the bowl of a blender and blitz until you have a smooth batter. Leave to stand for 5 minutes (doing this makes the pancakes light and fluffy).

Heat a non-stick frying pan over a medium heat and add a little oil (or cooking spray oil). Add the batter, one small ladleful per pancake (roughly 1–2 tablespoons) to the pan, leaving enough space between the pancakes so they don't touch, and cook until bubbles form and the edges are cooked, about 2 minutes. Flip the pancakes over with a spatula. Cook for another minute or so on the other side, then transfer to a plate. Repeat the process with the remaining batter.

If you don't want to serve as you go, preheat the oven to 120°C/fan 100°C/gas mark ½ and stack the pancakes in the oven as you cook them, placing a strip of greaseproof paper in between each one to stop them from sticking.

Serve the pancakes topped with your favourite toppings. Any leftovers can be wrapped in foil or cling film and kept in the fridge for up to 2 days or in the freezer for up to 3 months. To reheat, microwave on high for 15–20 seconds for 1 pancake and about 60 seconds for 5 pancakes.

NUTRITION per pancake | **119** cals | **5** g protein | **4** g fat (**1** g saturates) | **15** g carbs (**4** g total sugars) | **2** g fibre

Fruit and granola yogurt pot

. . . .

This highly nutritious breakfast takes seconds to put together. I like making it with
Greek-style soya yogurt alternative as it has roughly double the protein of other soya yogurt
alternatives. Berries are rich in polyphenols, which help reduce oxidative stress and inflammation,
and improve blood vessel function and blood flow. I have used a mixture of Black Forest
fruit (blackcurrants, cherries and blackberries) in this recipe but you can substitute any other
frozen berries, such as blackberries, strawberries or blueberries. Make up batches of
compote and keep in the fridge for up to five days.

SERVES 2

200 g frozen Black Forest fruit,
  plus a few extra for serving
2 tsp agave or maple syrup
  (optional)
2 tbsp Maple, Pecan and
  Cranberry Granola (p. 76) or
  your favourite shop-bought
  granola
400 g plain Greek-style soya
  yogurt alternative

Put the frozen berries into a small pan and cook on a low heat for
10 minutes until the juices are released. Turn up the heat and cook for
a further 5 minutes until the mixture has thickened. Stir in the agave
or maple syrup if you wish. Set aside to cool.

Divide the compote between 2 glass pots or jam jars. Scatter over
half the granola and add half the yogurt to each. Spoon on the remaining
compote, another layer of yogurt, then finish off with the rest of the
granola. Decorate with the reserved berries

NUTRITION per serving | **374** cals | **16** g protein | **14** g fat (**2** g saturates) | **41** g carbs (**16** g total sugars) | **9** g fibre

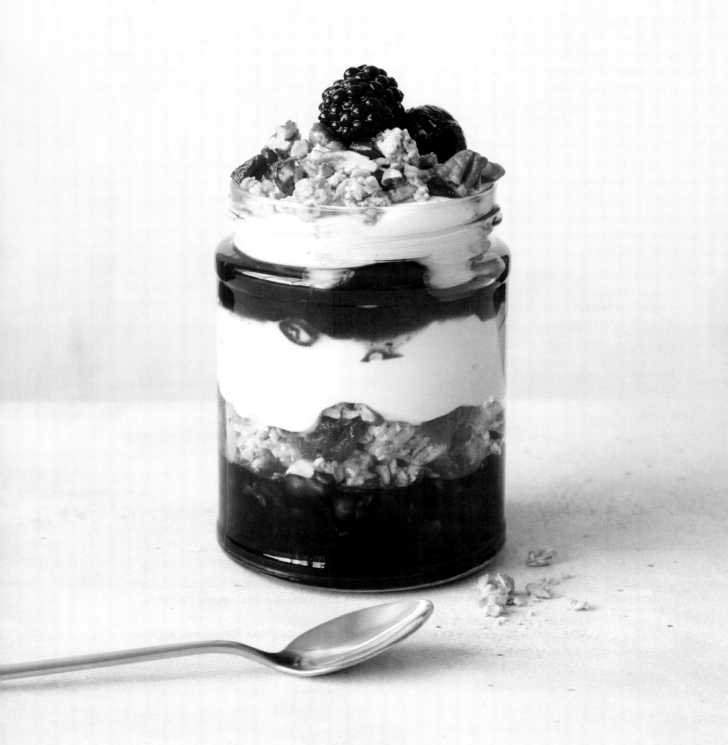

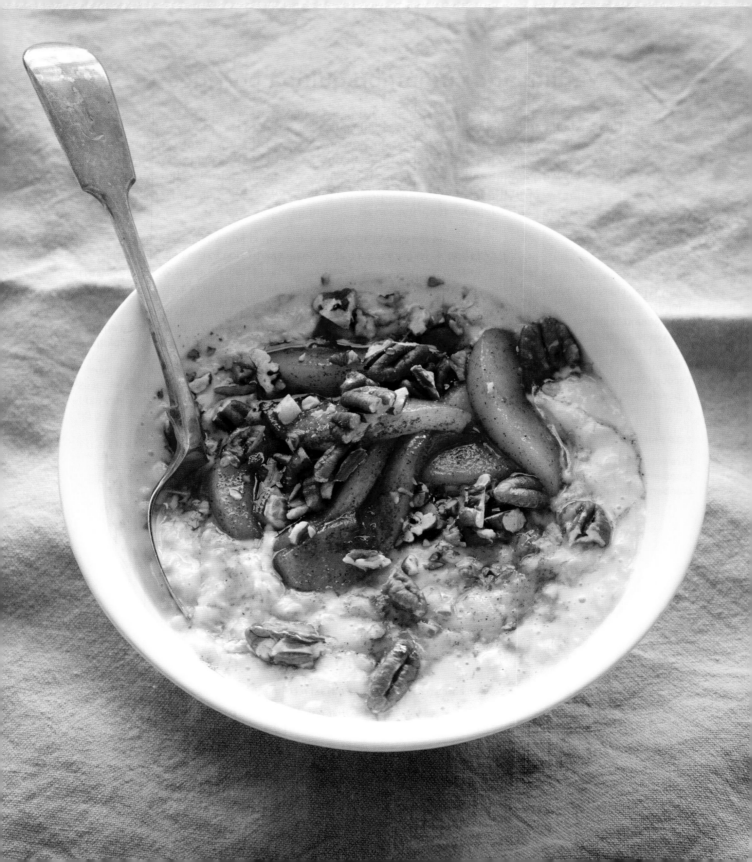

Spiced pear and pecan porridge

. . . .

Nothing is more warming and satisfying on a chilly morning than a bowl of steaming porridge. This protein-enriched version is ideal before a mid-morning or lunchtime workout. Topped with a layer of pears and pecans, it supplies 20 g of protein, the perfect amount for promoting muscle growth and recovery. You can substitute apple for the pear and use hazelnuts or walnuts instead of pecans.

SERVES 1

50 g jumbo oats
300 ml oat milk alternative, plus extra if needed (or use water) to thin
1 scoop (25 g) vanilla vegan protein powder

FOR THE TOPPING

1 pear, peeled, cored and sliced (e.g. Conference)
1–2 tsp maple syrup
¼ tsp ground cinnamon
2 tbsp water
1 tbsp toasted pecans (p. 57)

To make the topping, put the pear slices, maple syrup and cinnamon in a small saucepan with 2 tablespoons water. Bring to the boil, cover and simmer for 5–7 minutes.

Meanwhile, prepare the porridge by adding the oats and oat milk alternative to a separate saucepan. Bring to the boil, reduce the heat to a gentle simmer and cook, stirring often, for 4–5 minutes, until the porridge thickens.

Remove the porridge from the heat and stir in the protein powder. It will thicken further but if it is too thick, add extra oat milk alternative or water. Pour into a bowl and top with the syrupy pears and toasted pecans.

VARIATIONS

• *Blueberry and Coconut:* Make the porridge with coconut milk alternative and top with a handful of fresh blueberries and 1 tablespoon desiccated coconut.

• *Chocolate Banana:* Stir 1 teaspoon cocoa powder into the porridge, then top with banana slices and 1 tablespoon of cacao nibs or dark chocolate chips.

• *Apple Pie:* Cook the porridge with 1 grated apple, 1 tablespoon ground flaxseed, a handful of raisins and ¼ teaspoon cinnamon. Serve topped with flaked almonds.

• *Date and Apricot:* Cook the porridge with 2 chopped dried dates and 3 chopped dried apricots. Serve topped with 1 tablespoon toasted pumpkin seeds.

NUTRITION per serving | **421** cals | **21** g protein | **16** g fat (**1** g saturates) | **44** g carbs (**30** g total sugars) | **10** g fibre

Tofu scramble

· · · · · · · · · · · · · ·

I was a little sceptical before I tried this recipe but, trust me, it's a real game changer
if you miss having eggs! It is really tasty and has a wonderful texture. You can customise
it by adding your favourite spices (such as chilli powder or curry powder), fresh herbs
(such as basil, chives or parsley) or extra vegetables, such as baby spinach.
Tofu is high in protein and low in saturated fat.

SERVES 2

280 g firm tofu, drained
1 tbsp olive or rapeseed oil
4 spring onions, finely chopped
1 garlic clove, crushed
1 tsp turmeric
½ tsp smoked or sweet paprika
A pinch of nutritional yeast flakes
   (optional)
Salt and freshly ground black
   pepper, to taste

TO SERVE

Wholegrain or sourdough toast,
chilli flakes, avocado slices,
cherry tomatoes or mushrooms
(optional)

In a bowl, roughly mash the tofu using a fork.

Heat the oil in a non-stick frying pan over a high heat. Add the spring
onions and garlic and fry for 2–3 minutes until soft, then crumble in
the tofu, turmeric, paprika, nutritional yeast flakes and seasoning. Cook
for 2–3 minutes until you have a consistency similar to soft scrambled
eggs. Don't cook the scramble for too long otherwise it will become dry.
Serve on toast, topped with chilli flakes, avocado slices, tomatoes or
mushrooms – whatever you prefer.

NUTRITION
per serving* | **197** cals | **17** g protein | **13** g fat (**2** g saturates) | **2** g carbs (**2** g total sugars) | **1** g fibre

*without optional 'To serve' extras

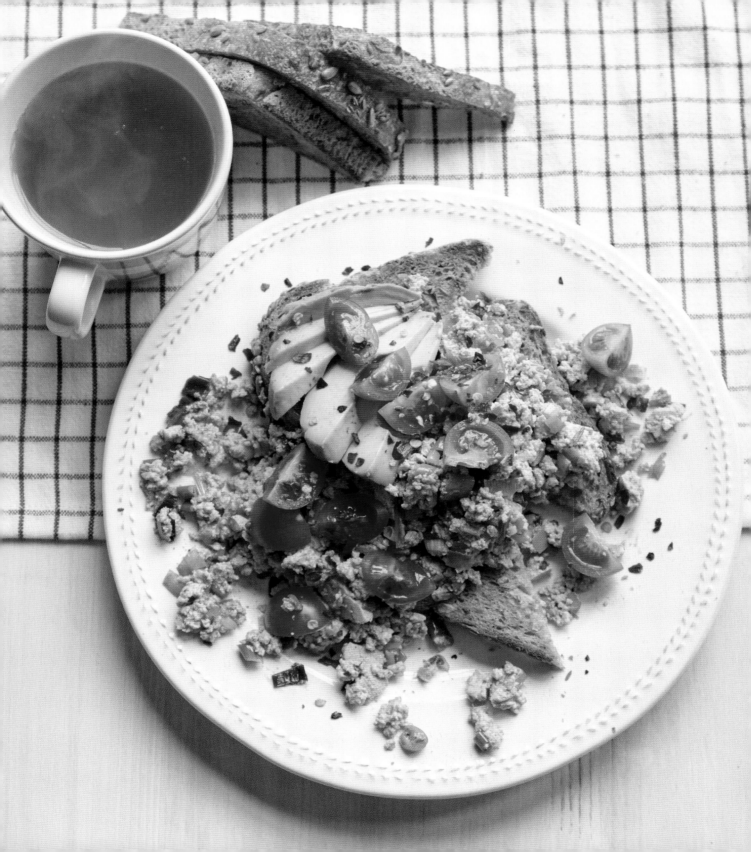

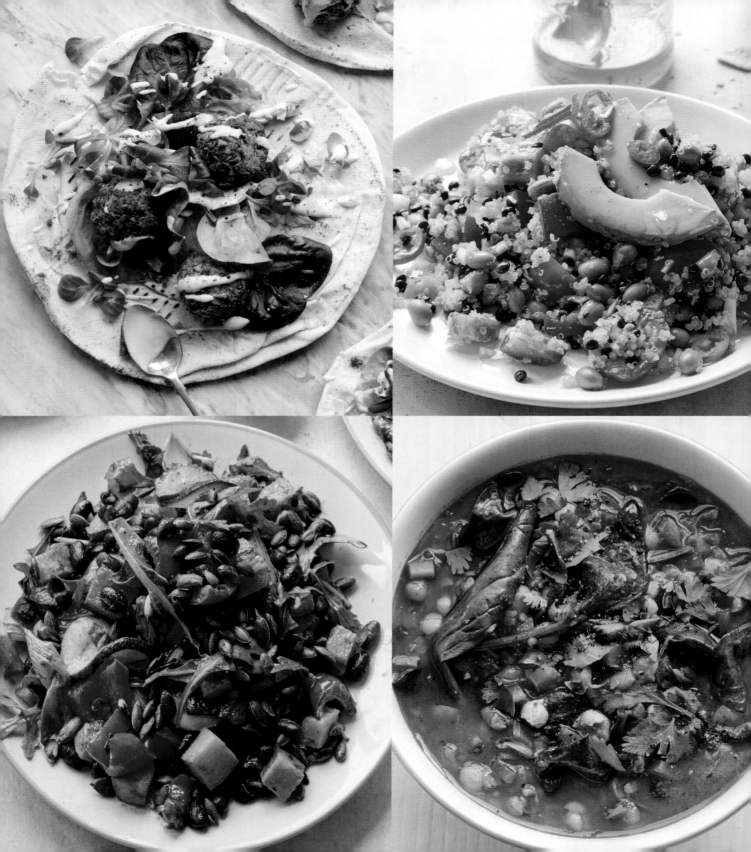

Light meals and salads

Clockwise from top left: Peri-peri pea falafel with tahini sauce;
Quinoa, edamame and avocado salad; Moroccan-spiced
chickpea soup; Black bean and sweet potato salad.

Beans and greens salad with pesto

....

This salad is perfect when you want something filling and nutritious! It combines creamy new potatoes with protein-rich cannellini beans, nutrient-packed green vegetables and heart-healthy pine nuts – giving you all the major groups in one meal. I have added tenderstem broccoli and spinach, both of which are rich in vitamin C and folate, but feel free to swap them for kale, rocket or sugar snap peas. Pomegranate seeds are also vitamin C-rich, while avocados and pine nuts both provide high levels of monounsaturated fats and vitamin E. Again, feel free to substitute other types of nuts or seeds.

SERVES 4

750 g new potatoes, halved
250 g tenderstem broccoli, halved
100 g vegan basil pesto (shop-bought or homemade, *see box*)
2 x 400 g cans cannellini beans, drained and rinsed
1 bunch spring onions, sliced
1 avocado, peeled, pitted and diced
A handful of baby spinach

TO SERVE

50 g pine nuts, toasted (p. 57)
50 g pomegranate seeds

Cook the potatoes in a large pan of boiling salted water for 15 minutes, adding the tenderstem broccoli for the final 4 minutes of cooking time. While the vegetables are cooking, make the pesto.

Drain the vegetables, place in a large serving bowl with the cannellini beans, spring onions, avocado, spinach and pesto; toss together well. Scatter over the pine nuts and pomegranate seeds and serve.

VEGAN BASIL PESTO

50 g fresh basil leaves
2 tbsp nutritional yeast flakes
25 g pine nuts
Juice of ½ lemon
1 garlic clove, crushed
125 ml olive oil
Salt, to taste

Place the ingredients in the bowl of a food processor and blend together until smooth. Season with salt to taste.

NUTRITION per serving | **571** cals | **20** g protein | **27** g fat (**3** g saturates) | **54** g carbs (**7** g total sugars) | **17** g fibre

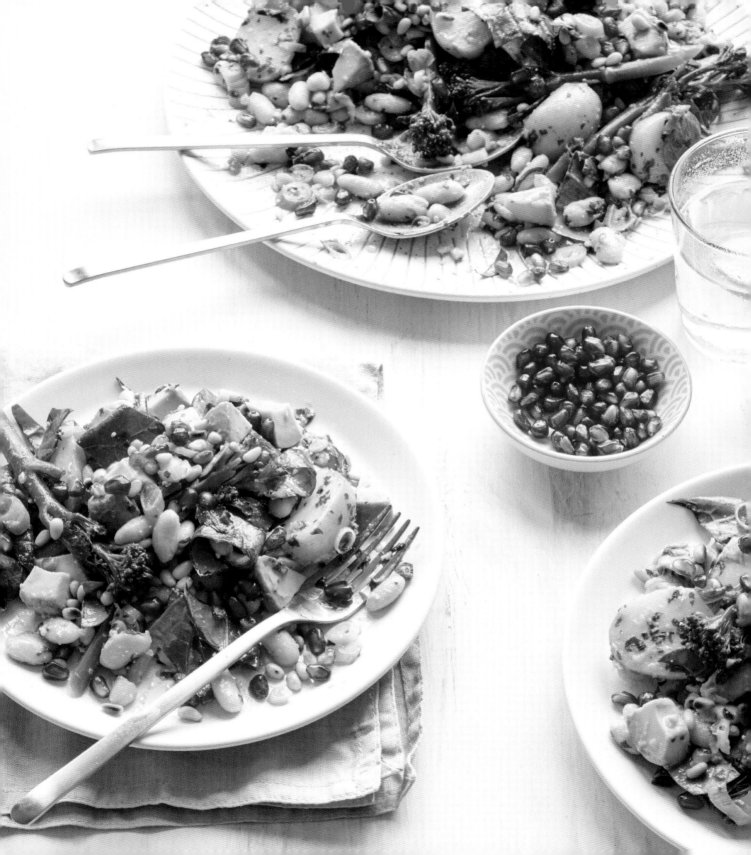

Black bean and rice buddha bowl

....

A buddha bowl is essentially a bowl of small portions of different foods, typically consisting of a grain (e.g. rice), a pulse (e.g. beans), plenty of vegetables and a dressing. It is so-called as it is usually eaten from a bowl with a wide top that signifies Buddha's belly! The combination of grains and beans provides the perfect balance of essential amino acids, as well as carbohydrate, healthy fats and a whole host of vitamins and minerals. The ingredients are flexible – add more or less of whatever you have on hand. You could use thinly sliced raw broccoli or cauliflower instead of the sugar snap peas or substitute roasted vegetables for any of the raw vegetables in this recipe. Assemble your ingredients in a big bowl, drizzle with dressing and you have a healthy, delicious meal ready to go.

SERVES 1

A handful of baby spinach, chopped romaine lettuce, or kale
125 g cooked brown rice, quinoa or bulgur wheat (or ½ x 250-g packet ready-bought)
½ x 400 g can (125 g drained weight) black beans (or chickpeas or any other type of beans)
1 carrot, grated
1–2 radishes, thinly sliced or 5–6 cherry tomatoes, cut in half
A handful of sugar snap peas, roughly chopped or thinly sliced broccoli florets
½ avocado, peeled, pitted and sliced
1 tbsp hummus (ready-bought or Chickpea Hummus, p. 188)
1–2 tbsp pumpkin, chia or sesame seeds, toasted (p. 57)
Extra virgin olive oil, lime juice, sea salt flakes and chilli flakes (optional)

Add a layer of baby spinach or other green vegetable to the bottom of your bowl, followed by a layer of cooked brown rice, quinoa or bulgur wheat. Top with black beans, grated carrot, radishes (or tomatoes), sugar snap peas, avocado and hummus. Sprinkle over the toasted seeds, then add a drizzle of extra virgin olive oil, a squeeze of lime and a sprinkle of sea salt flakes and chilli flakes, if liked.

| NUTRITION per serving | **650** cals | **24** g protein | **25** g fat (**4** g saturates) | **74** g carbs (**8** g total sugars) | **18** g fibre |

Lentil tabbouleh

· · · · · · · · · · · · ·

This simple salad made with ready-cooked puy lentils is full of Middle Eastern flavour. It provides 20 g protein, the perfect amount for muscle growth. The fresh herbs are rich sources of phytonutrients, while the red pepper and tomatoes provide plenty of vitamin C. I like to mix in pumpkin seeds, an excellent source of protein and alpha linolenic acid (ALA), plant-based omega-3 fats that support immunity and promote recovery. Swap for walnuts if you prefer.

SERVES 2

250 g pouch-cooked puy lentils*
4 spring onions, finely sliced
½ red pepper, deseeded and
    finely chopped
A handful of fresh flat-leaf
    parsley, finely chopped
A handful of fresh mint, finely
    chopped
125 g cherry tomatoes, halved
2 tbsp extra virgin olive oil
Juice of ½ lemon
2 tbsp pumpkin or walnut seeds,
    toasted (p. 57)
2 tbsp pomegranate seeds
Salt and freshly ground black
    pepper, to taste

Mix the lentils in a bowl with the spring onions, red pepper, herbs, cherry tomatoes, olive oil and lemon juice. Season with salt and freshly ground black pepper. Pile the tabbouleh into bowls and sprinkle over the pumpkin or walnut and pomegranate seeds.

*Alternatively use 100 g dried green or brown lentils. Rinse thoroughly, place in a pan with twice their volume of water (and a bay leaf, if you wish) and cook for 20–30 minutes or until tender.

NUTRITION per serving | **421** cals | **20** g protein | **21** g fat (**3** g saturates) | **33** g carbs (**8** g total sugars) | **13** g fibre

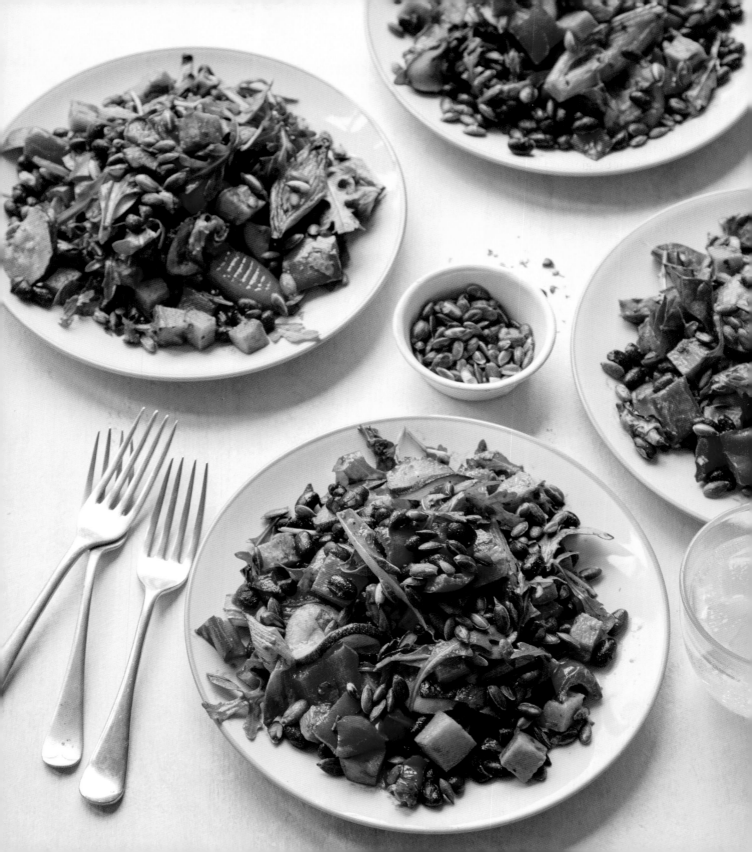

Black bean and sweet potato salad

. . . .

This colourful salad of black beans and sweet potatoes has long been a staple in my kitchen. Packed with protein, fibre, iron and antioxidant nutrients like beta-carotene, it's a brilliant recovery meal for vegan athletes. It's so customisable too – you can substitute butternut squash, aubergine or red onion for any of the veg in this recipe. It will keep for several days in the fridge so you can double the recipe to use for meals throughout the week.

SERVES 4

2 large, sweet potatoes (200 g each), washed and cut into 1-cm cubes
2 red peppers, deseeded and chopped
6 shallots, halved
3 tbsp light olive or rapeseed oil
1 tsp sweet paprika
2 courgettes, sliced
2 x 400 g cans black beans, drained and rinsed
A small handful of fresh coriander or parsley, chopped
Juice of 1 lime (or lemon)
100 g rocket, kale or baby spinach
75 g pumpkin seeds, toasted (p. 57)
Salt and freshly ground black pepper, to taste

Preheat the oven to 200°C/fan 180°C/gas mark 6.

Arrange the sweet potatoes, red peppers and shallots in a large roasting tin. Drizzle in 2 tablespoons of the oil, add the paprika, salt and freshly ground black pepper and toss so that the vegetables are well-coated. Roast in the oven for about 20 minutes, mix in the courgettes and continue cooking for a further 10 minutes until the vegetables are tender and starting to brown on the outside.

In a large bowl, combine the roasted vegetables with the beans, herbs, citrus juice, the remaining 1 tablespoon oil and the greens. Divide between four plates and scatter over the pumpkin seeds.

NUTRITION per serving | **481** cals | **20** g protein, **19** g fat (**3** g saturates) | **51** g carbs (**11** g total sugars) | **16** g fibre

Mexican bean and avocado tacos with tahini sauce

. . . .

These tasty tacos are packed with protein, fibre and essential fats. They contain three different sources of protein from red kidney beans, tortilla wraps and tahini, so you will be getting a perfect balance of essential amino acids. I have used toasted mini tortilla wraps instead of pre-fried, taco shells from supermarkets as it's much easier to keep the filling inside when you bite into them! You can substitute black or pinto beans for the red kidney beans.

SERVES 2

1 tbsp olive oil
½ red onion, finely chopped
1 red pepper, deseeded and
   chopped
1 tsp smoked sweet paprika
400 g can red kidney (or black
   or pinto) beans, drained
   and rinsed
200 g cherry tomatoes, halved
½ large avocado, peeled, pitted
   and chopped
75 g canned sweetcorn, drained
   and rinsed
Juice of ½ lime or lemon
A handful of fresh coriander,
   roughly chopped
4 mini tortilla wraps
Salt and freshly ground black
   pepper, to taste

FOR THE TAHINI SAUCE

2 tbsp tahini
1 tbsp lemon juice
1 tbsp water
A pinch of salt
1 small garlic clove, crushed

Heat the oil in a non-stick frying pan, add the onion and red pepper and fry over a medium heat for 2–3 minutes until softened. Add the smoked paprika and beans, season with salt and pepper and cook for a further 3 minutes.

In a bowl, combine the tomatoes, avocado, sweetcorn, citrus juice and fresh coriander to make a salsa.

To make the tahini sauce, add all the ingredients to a measuring jug and whisk until smooth. Add a little extra water if you prefer a thinner consistency.

Heat the tortillas one at a time in a dry frying pan for 15 seconds on each side or until lightly toasted. Keep them warm (a plate covered with a tea towel works very well).

To serve, divide the beans among the tortillas, then top with the salsa mixture and drizzle over the tahini sauce. Fold the tortillas over and serve.

| NUTRITION per serving | **599** cals | **20** g protein | **27** g fat (**5** g saturates) | **60** g carbs (**13** g total sugars) | **21** g fibre |

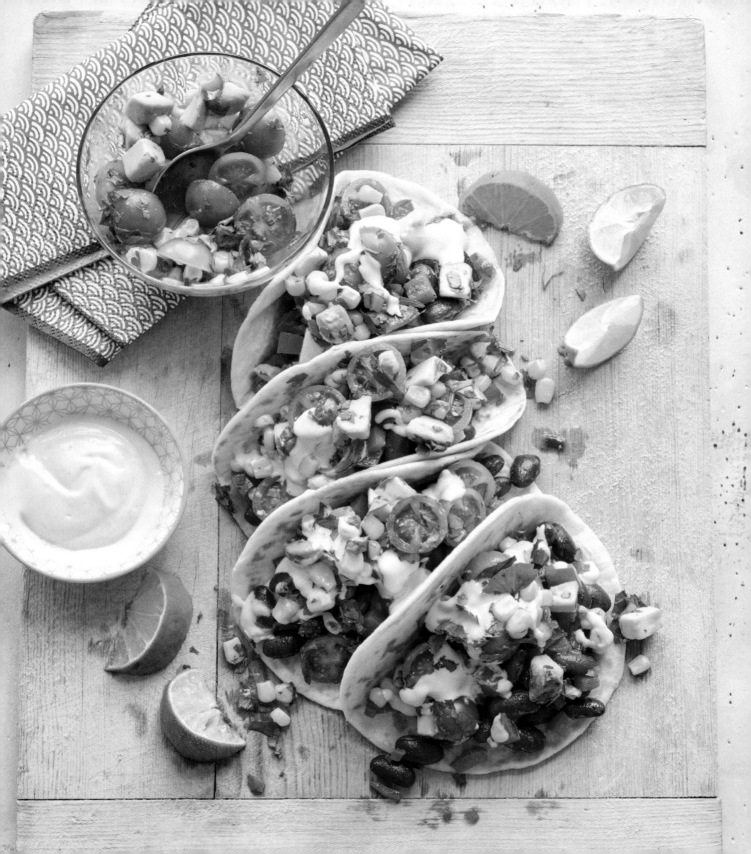

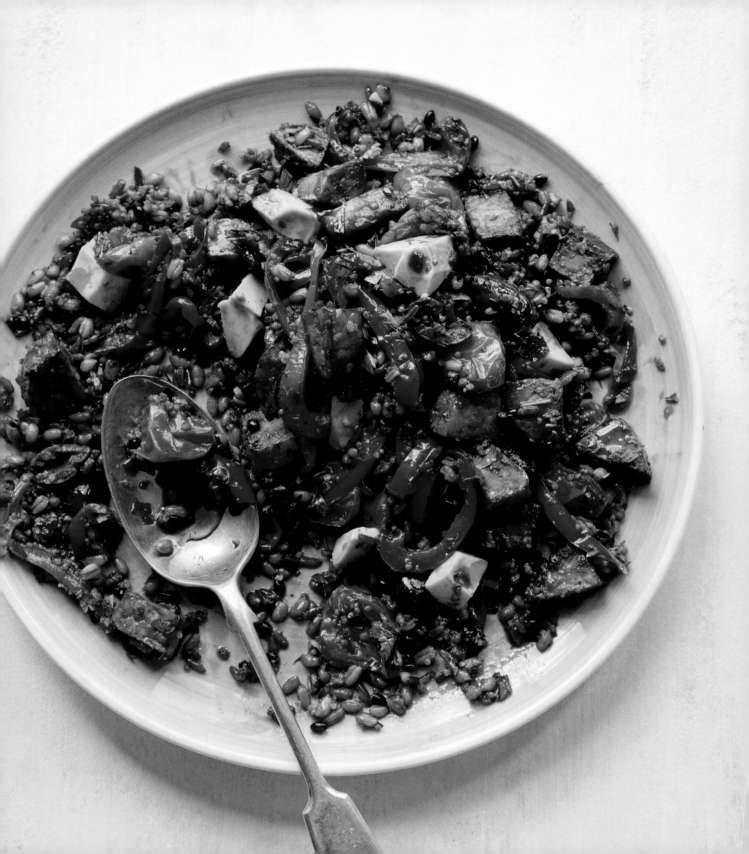

Mixed grain salad with crispy tempeh and harissa dressing

············

The base of this nutritious salad is cooked grains, which are excellent sources of fibre, carbohydrate, protein, B vitamins, iron and zinc. They are widely available in pouches from supermarkets, but you can cook any mixture of rice, bulgur or quinoa from scratch if you prefer. Tempeh, made from whole fermented soya beans, is rich in protein and provides a high concentration of all nine essential amino acids (*see also* p. 34). I like to flavour it with tamari (Japanese soy sauce) and nutritional yeast – this also gives it golden crispy edges when baked. Avocado and olives add healthy unsaturated fats, while the red peppers and tomatoes supply plenty of vitamin C.

SERVES 4

200 g tempeh
2 tbsp tamari (Japanese soy sauce) or soy sauce
1 tbsp nutritional yeast flakes
2 red peppers, deseeded and cut into strips
10 baby plum tomatoes, halved
2 garlic cloves, finely chopped
4 tbsp extra virgin olive oil
1 tbsp harissa paste
1 tsp agave or maple syrup
2 x 250-g pouches cooked mixed grains (e.g. rice, quinoa or bulgur wheat)
25 g black olives, pitted and halved
1 avocado, peeled, pitted and cubed
A small handful of flat-leaf parsley, finely chopped
Salt and freshly ground black pepper, to taste

Preheat the oven to 200°C /fan 180°C/gas mark 6.

Cut the tempeh into 2-cm cubes, add to a bowl and toss with the tamari or soy sauce and nutritional yeast flakes. Spread out on a lined baking tray, then bake for 25 minutes, tossing regularly.

Meanwhile, in a roasting tin, combine the pepper strips with the tomatoes, garlic and 2 tablespoons of the olive oil, then season with salt and freshly ground black pepper. Roast in the oven for 25 minutes, until the peppers are soft and just starting to char. Remove from the oven and allow to cool a little.

In a small bowl, whisk together the remaining olive oil, harissa paste and agave or maple syrup to make a dressing.

In a large serving bowl, combine the cooked grains, roasted vegetables, tempeh, olives, avocado, parsley and the dressing. Season with salt and freshly ground black pepper and toss well to ensure the dressing coats everything. Serve immediately.

NUTRITION per serving | **501** cals | **20** g protein | **24** g fat (**4** g saturates) | **46** g carbs (**6** g total sugars) | **12** g fibre

Moroccan-spiced chickpea soup

....

This simple, protein-packed soup is highly nutritious and easy to make. Chickpeas are high in fibre, particularly a type called oligosaccharides that are fermented by beneficial bacteria in the gut. They produce short-chain fatty acids (SCFAs) that improve immune function and benefit your health in so many ways, including post-exercise recovery.

SERVES 2

1 tbsp olive or rapeseed oil
1 small onion, finely chopped
1 carrot, finely chopped
1 celery stick, finely chopped
½ tsp ground cumin
½ tsp cinnamon
1 tsp harissa paste
2 tbsp tomato purée
400 ml vegetable stock
400 g can chickpeas, drained
    and rinsed
Juice of ½ lemon
50 g baby spinach
Salt and freshly ground black
    pepper, to taste

TO SERVE

Handful of fresh coriander,
    chopped
Toasted wholemeal pitta bread
    or flatbreads

Heat the oil in a large pan over a low heat and fry the onion, carrot and celery until the onion becomes translucent, about 5 minutes. Stir in the cumin, cinnamon, harissa paste, tomato purée, salt and freshly ground black pepper and cook for 1 minute, stirring.

Add the stock and chickpeas, bring to the boil and simmer for 5 minutes. Remove from the heat. Using a potato masher or hand blender, mash some of the soup in the pan. Stir in the lemon juice and spinach and let it cook in the heat of the soup for a couple of minutes until wilted. Adjust the seasoning, if necessary. Divide the soup between two bowls, sprinkle with coriander and serve with toasted pitta bread.

NUTRITION per serving	291 cals | 12 g protein | 11 g fat (1 g saturates) | 31 g carbs (11 g total sugars) | 12 g fibre
	Including 1 wholemeal pitta bread:
	489 cals | 20 g protein | 12 g fat (1 g saturates) | 68 g carbs (13 g total sugars) | 17 g fibre

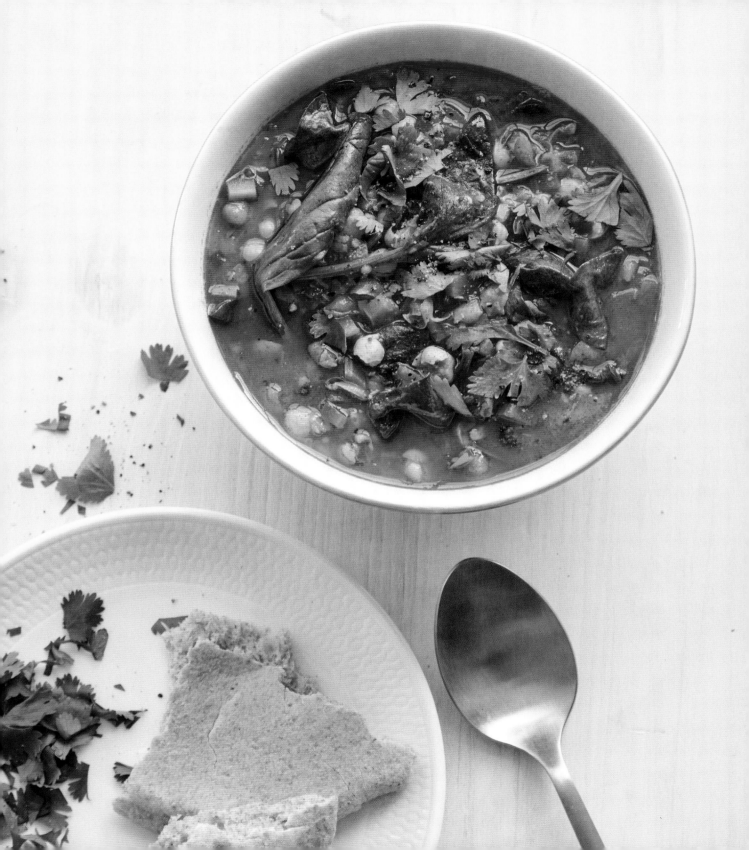

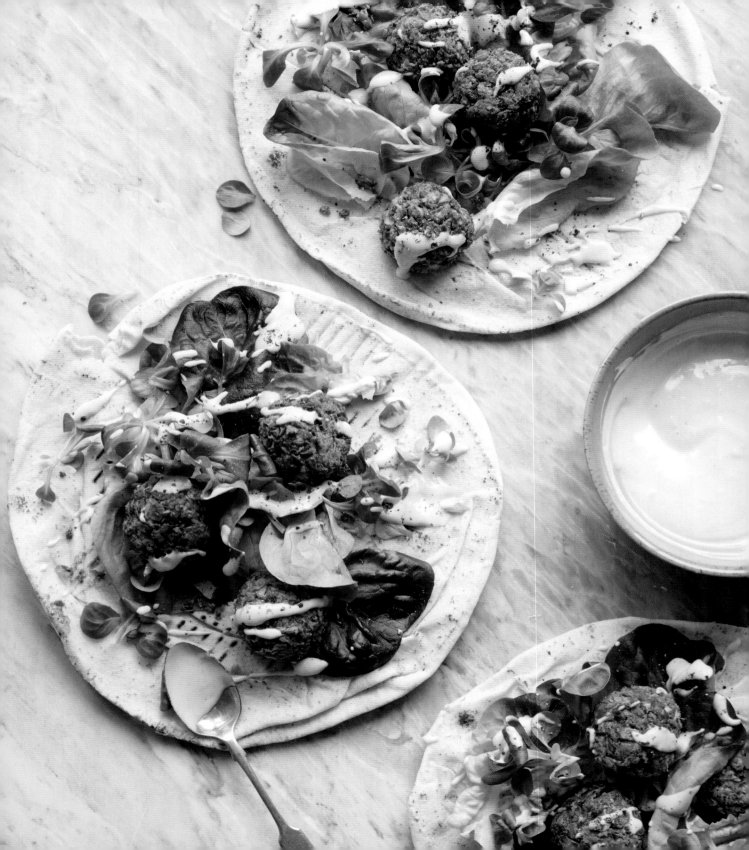

Peri-peri pea falafel with tahini sauce

....

These spicy falafels are perfect for lunchboxes and picnics. In this recipe, I have combined cooked frozen peas with canned chickpeas for a tasty twist on traditional falafels. The addition of the peas makes the falafels moist, so, unlike most baked falafel, they will not become dry or turn crumbly when you eat them. Served with flatbreads, salad and tahini sauce, you will be getting protein from four different sources, along with plenty of fibre, iron and vitamin C.

SERVES 4
MAKES APPROXIMATELY
12 FALAFELS

Oil for greasing
250 g frozen peas
400 g can chickpeas, drained
    and rinsed
½ small onion, roughly chopped
1 tbsp fresh coriander, chopped
A handful of fresh mint, chopped
2 garlic cloves, crushed
2 tsp cumin seeds (toasted in a
    dry frying pan) or 1 tsp ground
    cumin
2 tsp per-peri seasoning, or to
    taste
1 tbsp chickpea (gram) flour or
    plain flour mixed with 2 tbsp
    (30 ml) water, plus extra flour
    to coat
Salt and freshly ground black
    pepper, to taste

TAHINI SAUCE

2 tbsp tahini
2 tbsp lemon juice
1 garlic clove, crushed
5 tbsp cold water
Salt and freshly ground black
    pepper, to taste

Preheat the oven to 200°C/fan 180°C/gas mark 6. Meanwhile, lightly oil a baking sheet.

Boil the peas in salted water for 3 minutes; drain. Place the peas and chickpeas in the bowl of a blender or food processor and process for a few seconds. Add the onion, coriander, mint, garlic, cumin, peri-peri seasoning, chickpea (gram) or plain flour paste, salt and freshly ground black pepper. Process for a few seconds until roughly combined – it should still have a chunky texture otherwise it will turn into hummus.

Form the mixture into about 12 balls. Coat lightly with a little chickpea (gram) or plain flour. Place on the oiled baking sheet, brush with a little olive oil and bake for about 15–18 minutes until golden, turning once.

To make the sauce, combine the tahini, lemon juice and crushed garlic clove in a bowl along with the water and season with salt and pepper. Whisk until smooth.

Serve the falafels on grilled flatbreads, drizzled with the sauce and topped with leafy salad.

TO SERVE

4 flatbreads, grilled
Leafy salad

NUTRITION
per serving

3 falafels with tahini sauce:
245 cals | **12** g protein | **11** g fat (**2** g saturates) | **19** g carbs (**5** g total sugars) | **9** g fibre

3 falafels with tahini sauce and one flatbread:
546 cals | **20** g protein | **20** g fat (**3** g saturates) | **66** g carbs (**6** g total sugars) | **11** g fibre

Puy lentil salad with harissa-roasted cauliflower and walnuts

· · · · · · · · · · · · ·

This super-easy salad is full of contrasting flavours and textures and is a delicious way of boosting your fibre intake. The vibrant colour of harissa-roasted roasted cauliflower contrasts wonderfully with the dark lentils and is an excellent source of vitamin C. Puy lentils have the second-highest protein content of all pulses (after soya beans). I use ready-cooked puy lentils for speed, but dry lentils cooked for 30 minutes may also be used. The high vitamin C content of cauliflower, red peppers and tomatoes boosts the body's absorption of iron from the lentils.

PART 2 • RECIPES

SERVES 4

2 tbsp olive oil
2 tsp harissa paste, or to taste
1 medium cauliflower, divided
   into florets
2 red peppers, deseeded and
   cut into 2-cm strips
50 g walnuts
2 x 250 g packets ready-cooked
   puy lentils
100 g cherry tomatoes, halved
6 spring onions, sliced
100 g mixture of baby spinach
   and rocket
A handful of fresh mint, chopped
Salt and freshly ground black
   pepper, to taste

FOR THE DRESSING

2 tbsp olive oil
Juice of 1 lemon
Salt and freshly ground black
   pepper, to taste

TO SERVE

Plain soya yogurt alternative
   (optional)

Preheat the oven to 200°C/fan 180°C/gas mark 6.

Mix the olive oil with the harissa paste. Arrange the cauliflower and red peppers in a large roasting tin with the harissa paste mixture, salt and freshly ground black pepper. Toss so the vegetables are well coated, then roast in the oven for about 25 minutes until slightly charred on the outside. Put the walnuts on a separate baking tray and pop in the oven for the final 8 minutes of cooking time.

Meanwhile, make the dressing. Place the oil, lemon juice, salt and pepper in a small jar with a tight-fitting lid and shake well.

In a large bowl, combine the puy lentils with the dressing, tomato halves, spring onions, roasted vegetables, baby spinach and rocket. Scatter over the chopped mint and toasted walnuts. Serve with a spoonful of yogurt, if liked.

| NUTRITION per serving* | 472 cals | 22 g protein | 23 g fat (3 g saturates) | 36 g carbs (11 g total sugars) | 15 g fibre |

*without yogurt

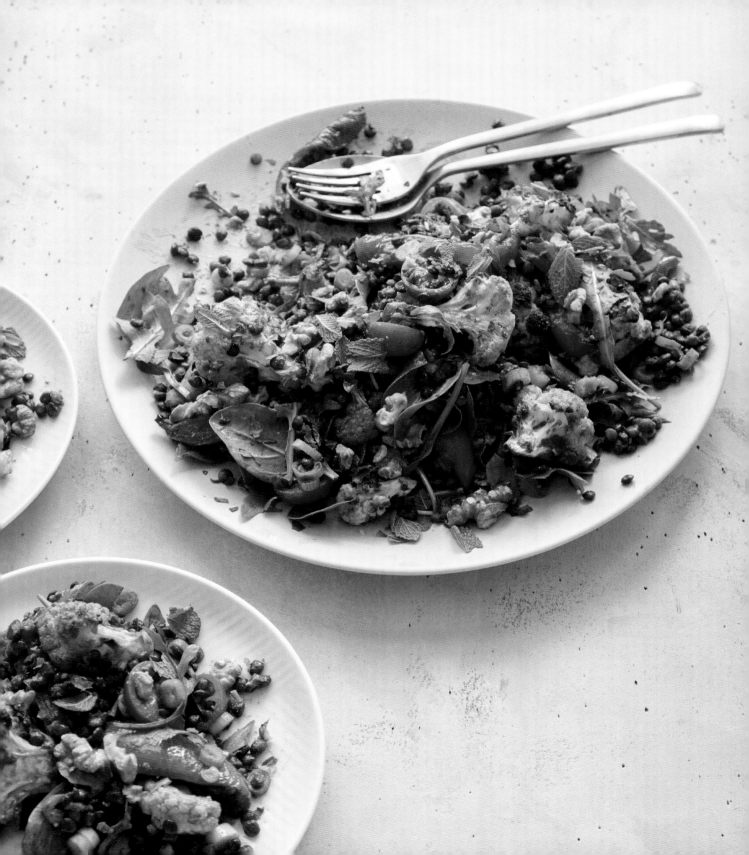

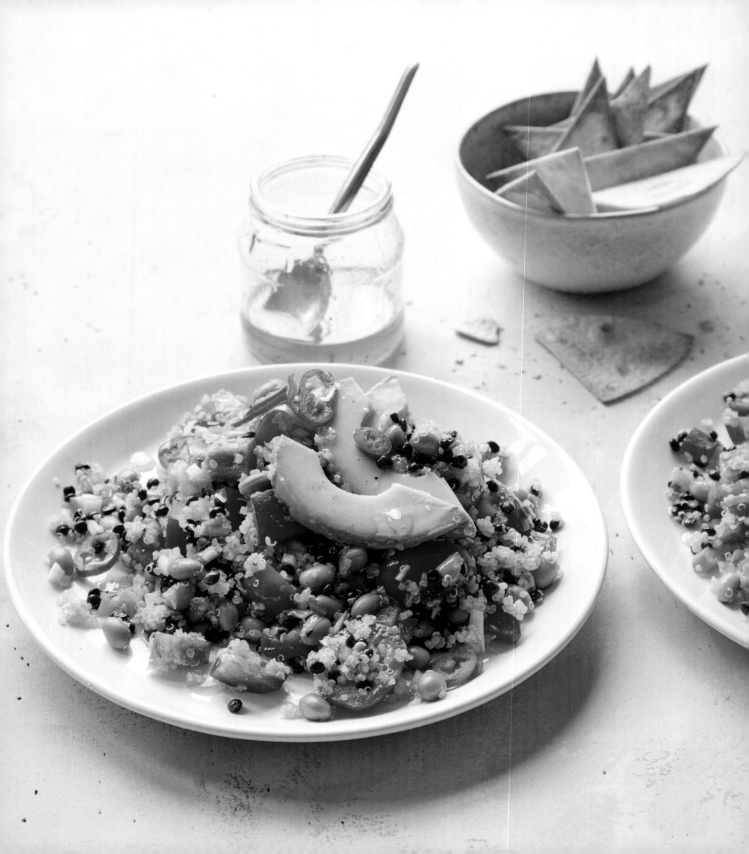

Quinoa, edamame and avocado salad with tortilla crisps

. . . .

This delicious salad includes three protein sources – quinoa, edamame beans and lentils – which together provide an excellent profile of amino acids, perfect for post-exercise recovery. The red peppers and tomatoes add lots of vitamin C, which helps increase the amount of iron that can be absorbed from the quinoa and lentils. I like to serve this salad with baked tortilla crisps, which are not only lower in fat than shop-bought, but so delicious and quick to make.

SERVES 4

125 g quinoa (or 250 g pouch-cooked quinoa)
250 g frozen edamame beans
250 g pouch-cooked Beluga lentils (or 400 g can Beluga lentils)
2 red peppers, deseeded and diced
About 8 spring onions, chopped
150 g baby plum tomatoes, halved

FOR THE DRESSING

2 tbsp olive or rapeseed oil
Juice of 1 lime
1 tsp honey
Salt and freshly ground black pepper, to taste

FOR THE TORTILLA CRISPS

2 corn or wheat tortillas
1 tbsp olive or rapeseed oil

TO SERVE

2 small avocados, peeled, pitted and sliced
1–2 red chillies, deseeded and thinly sliced

Preheat the oven to 200°C/fan 180°C/gas mark 6.

To make the tortilla crisps, brush both sides of the tortillas lightly with the oil, then cut into triangles. Arrange in a single layer on a baking sheet and bake for 8–10 minutes until crisp and golden (keep a close eye on them as they can burn quite quickly). Leave to cool.

Cook the quinoa in a large saucepan of boiling water according to the directions on the packet, adding the frozen edamame beans for the last 3 minutes of cooking. Drain in a colander, then tip into a large bowl. Mix with the lentils, red peppers, spring onions and tomatoes.

Make the dressing by shaking the oil, lime juice, honey and salt and pepper in a bottle or screw-top jar. Pour over the salad and toss well to combine. Spoon onto 4 plates and top with avocado slices and scatter with chillies. Serve with the tortilla crisps.

| NUTRITION per serving | **558** cals | **23** g protein | **26** g fat (**5** g saturates) | **50** g carbs (**9** g total sugars) | **14** g fibre |

Roasted squash and black bean tortillas

· · · · · · · · · · · · ·

These colourful tortillas are an exciting twist on open sandwiches and can be switched up according to what vegetables you have available. I have used butternut squash in this recipe, but you can swap for sweet potatoes or carrots (cut into batons). Butternut squash is rich in beta-carotene and vitamin C, while black beans are excellent sources of fibre and protein.

SERVES 2

¼ butternut squash (about 250 g), peeled, cut into 2-cm chunks
1 tbsp light olive or rapeseed oil
1 tsp ground cumin
½ tsp hot smoked paprika
2 wholemeal tortilla wraps
400 g can black beans, rinsed and drained
1 small red onion, thinly sliced

AVOCADO MASH

1 large avocado
Juice of ½ lemon
Salt and freshly ground black pepper, to taste

TO SERVE

2 tbsp plain Greek-style soya yogurt alternative

Preheat the oven to 200°C/fan 180°C/gas mark 6. Arrange the squash in a roasting tin and toss with the oil and spices, then roast for 20–25 minutes, stirring halfway, until golden.

Meanwhile, peel, pit and roughly mash the avocado in a bowl with the lemon juice, salt and freshly ground black pepper.

Toast the tortillas in a dry frying pan for 30 seconds on each side until warmed through. Arrange on plates, spread with mashed avocado, and top with the roasted squash and black beans. Scatter with onion slices and serve immediately with the yogurt to spoon over.

NUTRITION per serving | **572** cals | **20** g protein | **25** g fat (**4** g saturates) | **58** g carbs (**11** g total sugars) | **19** g fibre

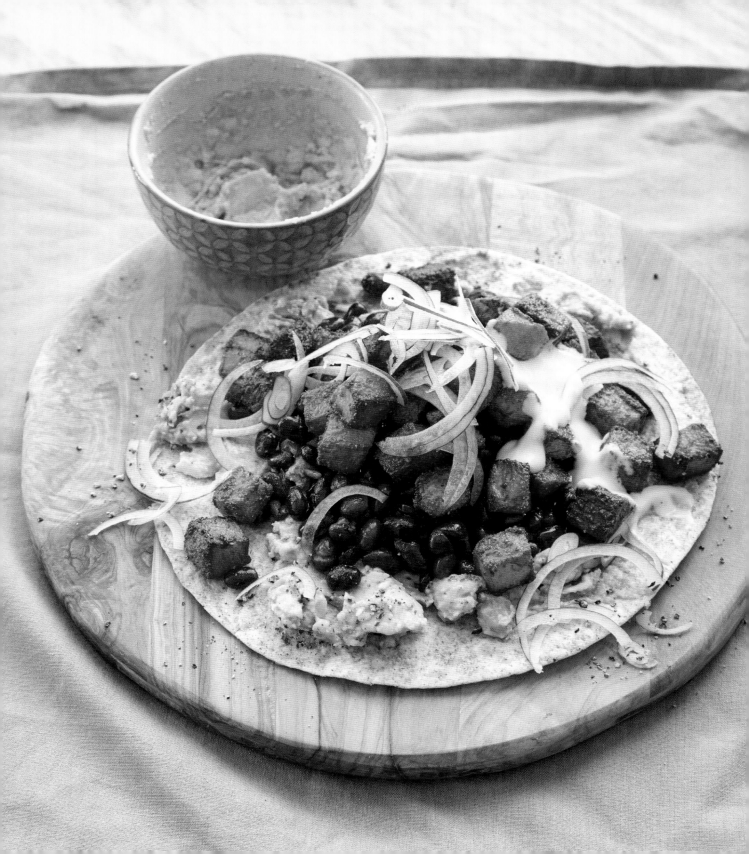

Sweet potato, beetroot and chickpea salad

· · · · · · · · · · · ·

This highly nutritious salad really ticks off all the food groups: carbohydrate, proteins, healthy fat, and fruit and vegetables. It also provides plenty of beta-carotene, vitamin E and vitamin C, powerful antioxidant nutrients that promote muscle recovery. Chickpeas are a brilliant source of fibre that nurtures the healthy microbes in the gut, which in turn helps reduce inflammation after intense exercise and supports immunity. Beetroot and salad leaves are rich in nitrates that raise nitric oxide levels in the body and improve both endurance and intermittent high-intensity exercise performance.

PART 2 • RECIPES

SERVES 4

2 large, sweet potatoes, peeled and cut into 1-cm cubes
1 red onion, finely sliced
1 tsp paprika
1 tsp ground cumin
1 tsp garlic granules
1 tbsp olive or rapeseed oil
2 x 400 g cans chickpeas, drained and rinsed
4 cooked whole beetroot, cut into wedges*
1 pear, peeled, cored and cubed
150 g mixed salad leaves, e.g. baby spinach, rocket or watercress
100 g pumpkin seeds, toasted (p. 57)
25 g dried cranberries (optional)
Salt and freshly ground black pepper, to taste

FOR THE DRESSING

1 tbsp balsamic vinegar
2 tbsp extra virgin olive oil

Preheat the oven to 180°C/fan 160°C/gas mark 4.

Meanwhile, arrange the sweet potato and red onion slices in a large roasting tin and sprinkle over the paprika, cumin, garlic granules, salt and freshly ground black pepper. Pour over 1 tablespoon oil and mix with your hands until the vegetables are well-coated. Make sure everything is spread out evenly. Roast in the oven for 30 minutes, taking out and stirring halfway through.

In a large bowl, combine the chickpeas, beetroot, pear and salad leaves. Once the sweet potatoes and onion are cooked, remove from the oven and allow to cool for a few minutes before adding to the salad bowl.

Make the dressing by whisking the balsamic vinegar and olive oil together. Pour over the salad, toss to combine, then scatter over the toasted pumpkin seeds and dried cranberries, if liked.

*Alternatively, use 4 raw beetroot cut into wedges. Toss with an extra 1 tablespoon oil in the same roasting tin as the sweet potatoes, keeping them separate as much as possible. Roast in the oven at the same temperature for 30 minutes.

NUTRITION per serving | **556** cals | **20** g protein | **24** g fat (**3** g saturates) | **57** g carbs (**22** g total sugars) | **16** g fibre

Teriyaki tempeh noodle bowl

. . . .

Tempeh is a quick and easy way to add lots of protein to your meal. It has an amazing texture – it's much firmer than tofu as it's made using the whole soya bean. Once fried, the tempeh becomes crispy and when added to the sweet and salty teriyaki sauce, it absorbs it like a sponge. In this recipe, it is served with stir-fried vegetables over noodles, but you can substitute raw vegetables if you wish. Either way, this dish is a super-tasty way of getting lots of vitamin C, beta-carotene, fibre and folate.

SERVES 2

100 g tempeh
2 tbsp light olive or rapeseed oil
1 onion, roughly diced
1 tsp grated garlic
2 tsp grated fresh root ginger
1 red pepper, deseeded and
   roughly diced
150 g tenderstem broccoli
6–8 baby corn

FOR THE TERIYAKI SAUCE

1 tbsp cornflour mixed with
   2 tbsp water
4 tbsp light soy sauce
1 tbsp rice wine vinegar
1 garlic clove, crushed
1 tsp fresh root ginger, grated
2 tbsp maple syrup or brown
   sugar

TO SERVE

2 nests (2 x 50 g) of soba noodles
1 tbsp toasted sesame seeds
   (p. 57)

First, cook the noodles according to the packet instructions. Drain and return to pan to keep warm.

Cut the tempeh into triangles. Heat 1 tablespoon of the oil in a non-stick frying pan over a medium-high heat and fry the tempeh until golden brown on all sides. Transfer to paper towels to drain.

Combine the teriyaki sauce ingredients in a bowl, mix well and set to one side.

Heat the remaining oil in a wok over a medium-high heat, add the onion, garlic and ginger and fry until fragrant and the onion is translucent.

Add the remaining vegetables and cooked tempeh and stir-fry for 3–4 minutes. Add the sauce mixture, bring to the boil and simmer for 1 minute.

Serve the vegetable mixture on top of the cooked noodles, sprinkled with toasted sesame seeds.

NUTRITION per serving* | **584** cals | **25** g protein | **21** g fat (**3** g saturates) | **68** g carbs (**23** g total sugars) | **13** g fibre

*including 1 nest of noodles

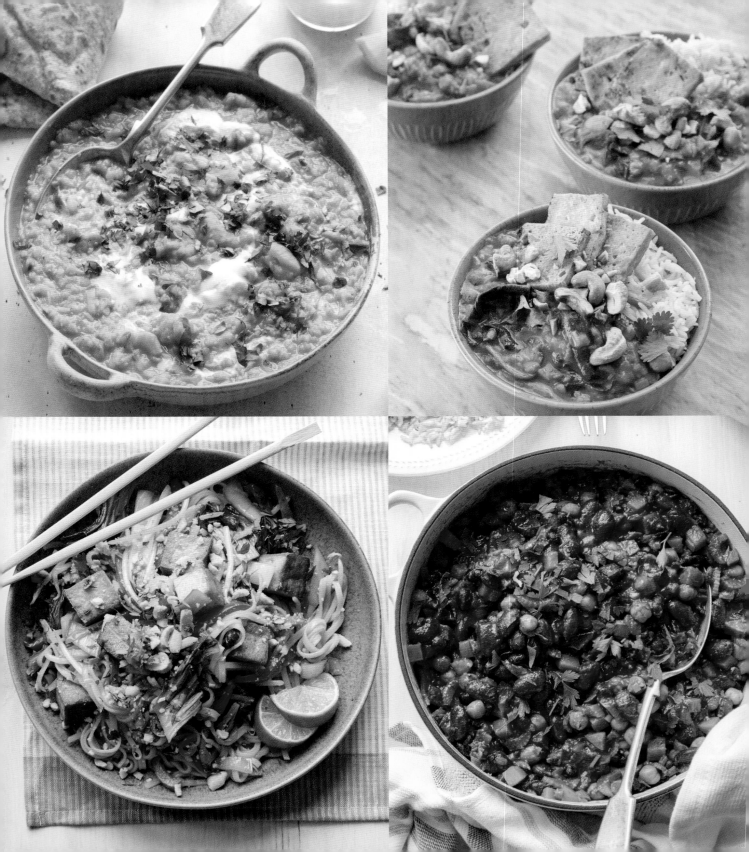

One-pot dishes

CHAPTER 11

Clockwise from top left: Red lentil dal; Tomato and coconut dal with crispy tofu and cashews; Three-bean chilli with cashew cream; Pad thai with crispy tofu.

Aubergine, chickpea and harissa traybake with a yogurt and mint sauce

. . . .

This low-effort traybake is a great make-ahead dish that will keep in the fridge (for up to three days) to reheat when needed. The heat of the harissa-spiced aubergines is balanced beautifully by the cool yogurt and mint sauce. Swap the chickpeas for canned green lentils or cannellini beans, if you prefer. It is high in fibre, protein, iron and vitamin C.

SERVES 4

2 tbsp olive or rapeseed oil

1 onion, thinly sliced

2 aubergines, cut into 2-cm cubes

2 tbsp harissa paste (or to taste)

400 g cherry tomatoes (or 400 g canned cherry tomatoes)

2 x 400 g cans chickpeas, drained and rinsed

Salt and freshly ground black pepper, to taste

FOR THE YOGURT AND MINT SAUCE

½ cucumber

500 g plain Greek-style soya yogurt alternative

2 tbsp fresh mint, finely chopped

TO SERVE

Toasted wholemeal flatbreads or pitta breads

Preheat the oven to 220°C/fan 200°C/gas mark 7. Pour the oil into a large roasting tin and heat in the oven for 5 minutes (this prevents the aubergines from soaking up too much oil), then add the onion, aubergines and harissa paste, and season with salt and freshly ground black pepper. Mix together, then roast for 30 minutes, stirring halfway through to make sure they cook evenly.

Add the tomatoes to the tray, then return to the oven for a further 15 minutes. Stir in the chickpeas and return to the oven for a final 15 minutes.

Meanwhile, grate the cucumber. Tip into a bowl and mix with the yogurt and mint.

When the traybake is ready, give it a good stir and adjust the seasoning, if necessary. Serve with the yogurt and mint sauce and toasted flatbreads or pitta breads.

NUTRITION per serving	375 cals	20 g protein	15 g fat (2 g saturates)	33 g carbs (13 g total sugars)	15 g fibre
	Including 1 pitta bread:				
	534 cals	25 g protein	16 g fat (2 g saturates)	63 g carbs (15 g total sugars)	20 g fibre

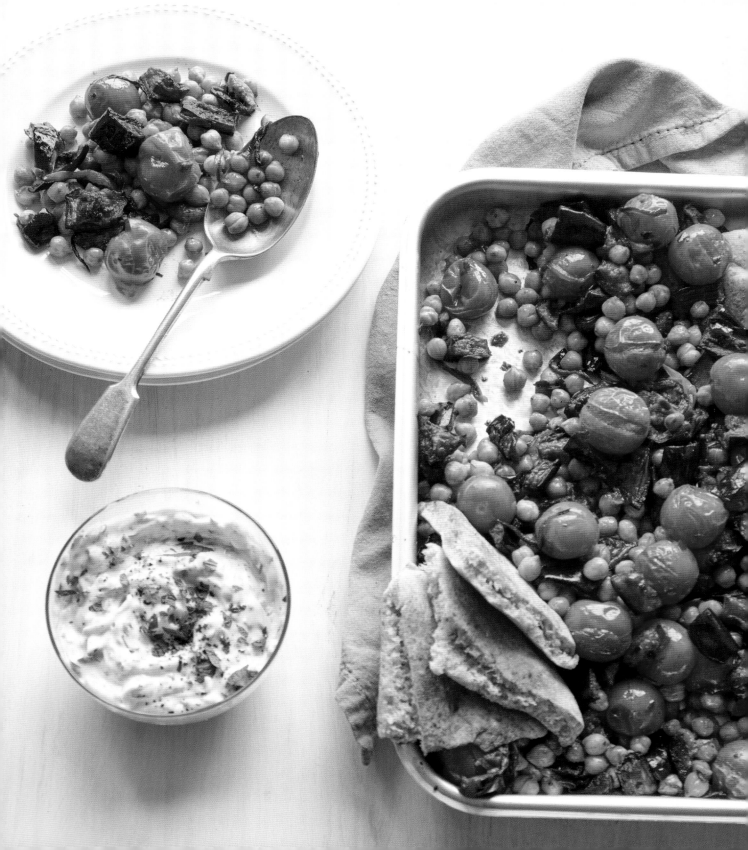

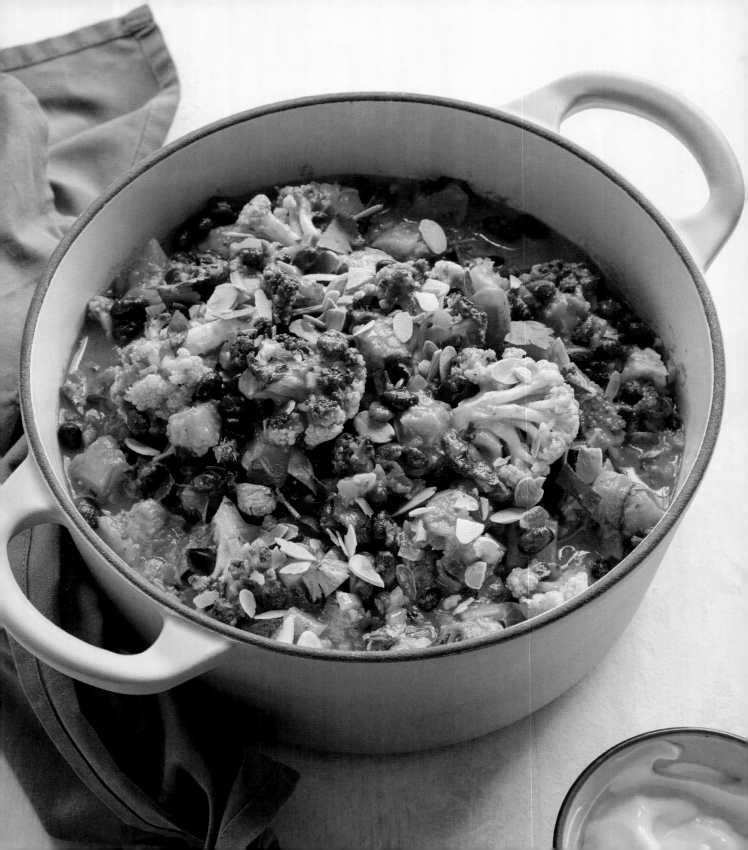

Black bean, butternut and cauliflower curry

. . . .

This tasty curry provides a perfect balance of carbohydrate and protein, along with high levels of phytonutrients that help promote muscle adaptation. Black beans are rich in protein and contain plenty of prebiotic fibre that provides food for your 'good' gut bacteria, helping them grow and thrive. Roasting the vegetables before adding to the curry sauce intensifies the flavour. It also means that while they are cooking, you can prepare the sauce and stir them in at the end, thus saving overall cooking time.

SERVES 4

½ butternut squash
  (approximately 500 g), peeled
  and cut into 1-cm cubes
1 small cauliflower (approximately
  600 g), cut into florets
2 tbsp light olive or rapeseed oil
1 onion, finely chopped
1 tsp cumin seeds
2–3 garlic cloves, crushed
2–3 cm piece fresh root ginger,
  peeled and grated or finely
  chopped
½ fresh red chilli, deseeded and
  finely chopped, or to taste
1 tsp ground coriander
½ tsp ground turmeric
½ tsp sweet paprika
2 tsp garam masala
200 g canned chopped tomatoes
250 ml water
200 ml canned coconut milk
2 x 400 g cans black beans,
  drained and rinsed
A large handful of fresh coriander,
  chopped
Juice of ½ lemon
Salt and freshly ground black
  pepper, to taste

Preheat the oven to 200°C/fan 180°C/gas mark 6. Place the prepared butternut squash and cauliflower on a baking tray and sprinkle over a little salt and pepper. Add 1 tablespoon of the oil and toss so all vegetables are well-coated. Roast in the oven for 20–25 minutes.

Meanwhile, heat the remaining oil in a large pan over a low to moderate heat. Add the onion and fry for 3–4 minutes until softened. Add the cumin seeds, garlic, ginger and chilli and fry for 1 minute. Stir in the remaining spices and fry for a further 1 minute.

Add the canned tomatoes, water, coconut milk and beans. Bring to the boil, then reduce the heat and simmer for 10 minutes.

Stir in the roasted vegetables and heat through. Add the coriander and lemon juice and season to taste. Scatter over the flaked toasted almonds and serve with a spoonful of yogurt alternative.

TO SERVE

50 g flaked almonds, toasted
  (p. 57)
4 tbsp plain Greek-style yogurt
  alternative

NUTRITION per serving* | **518** cals | **23** g protein | **24** g fat (**9** g saturates) | **44** g carbs (**15** g total sugars) | **16** g fibre

*including 1 tablespoon yogurt alternative

Black pepper tofu with pak choi and cashews

·············

If you've been searching for new ways of adding tofu to your diet, then this easy Vietnamese-inspired traybake is the one for you! It is packed with flavour, high in protein and a brilliant way of incorporating green vegetables in your diet. Everything is baked in one tray and served with a delicious peanut sauce. You can substitute kale or spinach for the pak choi (Chinese cabbage) or use almonds instead of cashews if you prefer.

SERVES 4

450 g firm smoked or marinated tofu, cut into 2-cm cubes
200 g chestnut mushrooms
175 g baby corn
2 tbsp sesame or rapeseed oil
2 garlic cloves, crushed
5-cm piece fresh root ginger, peeled and grated
400 g pak choi (Chinese cabbage), thinly sliced
50 g cashew nuts or almonds
Salt and freshly ground black pepper, to taste

FOR THE PEANUT SAUCE

100 g crunchy peanut butter
Finely grated zest and juice of 1 lime
2 tbsp soy sauce
2 tbsp rice wine vinegar
½–1 red chilli, deseeded and finely chopped
2-cm piece fresh root ginger, peeled and grated
1 garlic clove, crushed

TO SERVE

4 spring onions, finely sliced
200 g wholewheat or plain noodles (egg-free), cooked according to packet instructions

Preheat the oven to 220°C/fan 200°C/gas mark 7.

Arrange the tofu, mushrooms and baby corn in a large roasting tin, then mix in the oil, garlic, ginger, salt and freshly ground black pepper. Roast in the oven for 20 minutes.

Add the pak choi and the cashew nuts. Return to the oven for a further 15 minutes until the tofu is crisp and golden brown and the greens have wilted.

Meanwhile, whisk together the peanut sauce ingredients in a bowl and pour over as soon as the dish comes out of the oven.

Sprinkle with spring onions and serve with cooked noodles.

NUTRITION per serving | **492** cals | **31** g protein | **34** g fat (**6** g saturates) | **12** g carbs (**6** g total sugars) | **8** g fibre
Including 50 g (dry weight) wholewheat noodles:
670 cals | **37** g protein | **35** g fat (**6** g saturates) | **46** g carbs (**6** g total sugars) | **12** g fibre

Butter bean and butternut squash ragout with yogurt

· · · · · · · · · · · ·

A ragout is a slow-cooked, French-style chunky stew that is incredibly delicious and satisfying. This vegan version made with butter beans and vegetables is rich in protein, fibre, iron and antioxidant vitamins; one serving provides your entire daily requirement for vitamins A (as beta-carotene), C and E. You can substitute borlotti or cannellini beans for the butter beans and add mushrooms or any other vegetables you have handy.

SERVES 2

1 tbsp light olive or rapeseed oil
1 small onion, finely chopped
1 green or red pepper, deseeded and sliced
1 yellow pepper, deseeded and sliced
2 garlic cloves, crushed
1 tsp sweet paprika
1 tsp dried Italian herbs
¼ tsp cayenne pepper, or to taste
¼ butternut squash (approximately 250 g), peeled and cut into 1-cm cubes
400 g can butter beans, drained and rinsed
400 g can chopped tomatoes
2 tbsp tomato purée
250 ml vegetable stock or water
A handful of fresh parsley, chopped
4 tbsp plain Greek-style soya yogurt alternative
Salt and freshly ground black pepper, to taste

TO SERVE

2 medium jacket potatoes

Heat the oil in a large non-stick pan over a medium heat. Add the onion and peppers and fry for 3–4 minutes, then add the garlic, paprika, herbs, cayenne pepper and a generous pinch of salt and freshly ground black pepper. Continue cooking for 1 minute. Add the butternut squash and cook for a further 2–3 minutes.

Add the remaining ingredients apart from the parsley and yogurt. Stir and bring to the boil. Reduce the heat, cover with a lid and simmer for 15 minutes, stirring occasionally and adding a little water if necessary, until the vegetables are tender. Stir in most of the parsley.

Serve in bowls, topped with a spoonful of yogurt, scattering over the remaining parsley.

NUTRITION per serving	**401** cals	**20** g protein	**11** g fat (**2** g saturates)	**47** g carbs (**27** g total sugars)	**19** g fibre
	Including 1 medium jacket potato:				
	494 cals	**22** g protein	**11** g fat (**2** g saturates)	**66** g carbs (**28** g total sugars)	**21** g fibre

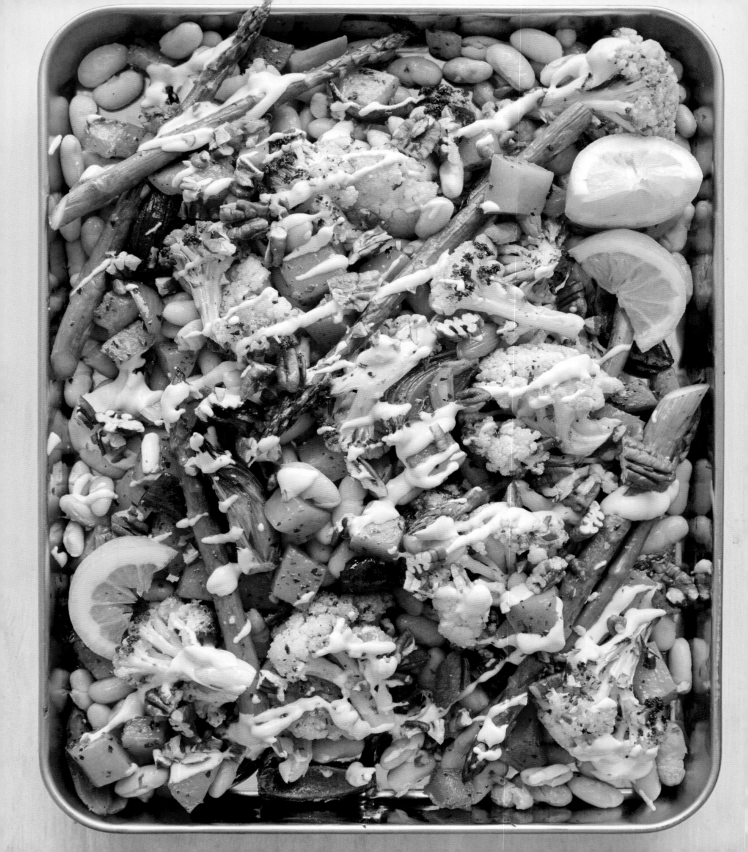

Cannellini bean, cauliflower and squash traybake

···········

This easy traybake is a tasty way to gets lots of colourful veg into your meal and the leftovers make a perfect lunch the next day. It includes three different protein sources – cannellini beans, pecans and tahini – ensuring a full complement of amino acids to support muscle recovery. Asparagus gives you plenty of inulin (prebiotic fibre), which helps your 'good' gut bacteria thrive. Pecans also supply plant-based omega-3s, which are essential for healthy cell membranes and brain function. You can substitute canned black or green lentils, chickpeas or black beans for the cannellini beans.

SERVES 4

½ butternut squash
   (approximately 500 g), peeled
   and cut into 1-cm cubes
1 cauliflower, divided into florets
2 red onions, cut into wedges
2 garlic cloves, crushed
2 tsp dried Italian herbs (or
   thyme)
3 tbsp extra virgin olive oil
2 x 400 g cans cannellini beans,
   drained and rinsed
125 g asparagus, cut into 5-cm
   lengths
Salt and freshly ground black
   pepper, to taste

TAHINI SAUCE

4 tbsp tahini
Juice of 1 lemon
1 tbsp Dijon mustard
1 tsp maple syrup
4 tablespoons water
75 g pecans, roughly chopped
Salt and freshly ground black
   pepper, to taste

Preheat the oven to 200°C/fan 180°C/gas mark 6.

Arrange the squash, cauliflower and red onions in a large roasting tin. Season with salt and pepper, sprinkle with the garlic and Italian herbs or thyme, then drizzle with olive oil. Toss lightly so all the vegetables are well-coated in oil, then roast for 25 minutes.

Remove the roasting tin from the oven. Add the cannellini beans and asparagus to the roasting tin. Return to the oven and roast for a further 5 minutes.

Meanwhile, prepare the tahini sauce. Combine the tahini with 1 tablespoon of the lemon juice, the mustard, maple syrup and 4 tablespoons water in a small mixing bowl until smooth and runny (adding a little more water, as necessary). Taste and season.

Remove the roasting tin from the oven and squeeze the rest of the lemon juice on top. Drizzle the tahini dressing around the tin and scatter over the pecans.

NUTRITION
per serving | **598** cals | **23** g protein | **33** g fat (**4** g saturates) | **44** g carbs (**18** g total sugars) | **19** g fibre

Chickpea and butternut squash tagine

....

A tagine is basically a slow-cooked stew that originated in Morocco. It is flavoured with fragrant spices and traditionally cooked in a tall, conical tagine. This vegan version made with chickpeas and served with couscous provides an excellent balance of essential amino acids that promote muscle recovery. Plus, it is a rich source of fibre, B vitamins and beta-carotene, an antioxidant vitamin that protects against cell damage during exercise. Spinach and dried apricots both add plenty of iron, while almonds supply vitamin E. Ras el hanout, a blend of paprika, cumin, coriander, chilli, cinnamon, black pepper, cardamom and rose petal, is widely available from supermarkets and gives the tagine a wonderful aromatic flavour.

SERVES 4

2 tbsp light olive or rapeseed oil
1 onion, finely chopped
2 garlic cloves, crushed
2-cm piece fresh root ginger, peeled and finely chopped
1 tsp ras el hanout or harissa paste
½ tsp ground cumin
½ tsp ground coriander
½ tsp ground cinnamon
½ butternut squash (approximately 500 g), peeled, deseeded and cut into 1-cm chunks
400 g can chopped tomatoes
2 x 400 g cans chickpeas, drained and rinsed
75 g dried ready-to-eat apricots, roughly chopped
Juice of 1 lemon
50 g fresh spinach
Salt and freshly ground black pepper, to taste

TO SERVE

50 g flaked almonds, toasted (p. 57)
A small handful of fresh coriander, chopped
200 g couscous, cooked according to packet instructions

Heat the oil in a large pan over a medium heat and cook the onion for 3 minutes until translucent. Add the garlic, ginger, ras el hanout (or harissa paste), cumin, coriander and cinnamon. Stir well and cook for 1 minute. Add the butternut squash, tomatoes, chickpeas and dried apricots and top up with enough hot water to just cover the vegetables.

Bring to the boil, then turn down the heat and simmer for 20–25 minutes until the vegetables are tender. Add the lemon juice and spinach, stirring it in until just wilted. Season with salt and freshly ground black pepper.

Scatter over the flaked almonds and chopped coriander and serve with cooked couscous.

NUTRITION per serving | **413** cals | **16** g protein | **17** g fat (**2** g saturates) | **43** g carbs (**19** g total sugars) | **14** g fibre

Including 50 g (dry weight) couscous:
603 cals | **23** g protein | **18** g fat (**2** g saturates) | **81** g carbs (**20** g total sugars) | **16** g fibre

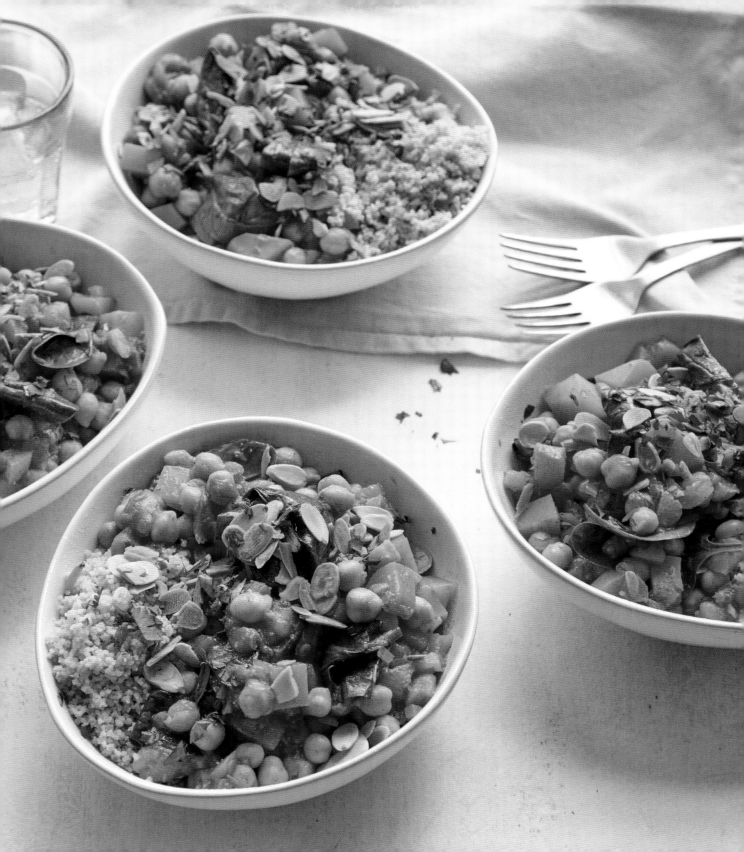

Cauliflower and butter bean curry with almonds

．．．．．．．．．．．．．．

Cauliflower is a great base for curries: it soaks up flavours, adds a great texture
and is a fantastic source of vitamin C – a quarter of a small head provides your entire daily
requirement. I have used butter beans in this recipe, but you can substitute red kidney beans,
chickpeas or whatever variety you fancy. A few dried apricots gives a subtle sweetness
to the sauce, while spinach adds iron and vibrant colour.

118

SERVES 2

1 tbsp light olive or rapeseed oil
1 small onion, chopped
2 garlic cloves, crushed
1-cm piece fresh root ginger,
    grated
1 tsp each cumin, coriander
    and garam masala, plus ½ tsp
    turmeric or 1 tbsp medium
    curry paste
½ small cauliflower, broken into
    florets
200 g canned chopped tomatoes
400 g can butter beans, drained
    and rinsed
4–5 dried apricots, chopped
200 ml water
50 g baby spinach
A small handful of fresh coriander,
    chopped
25 g flaked toasted almonds
    (p. 57)
Salt and freshly ground black
    pepper, to taste

TO SERVE

100 g basmati rice, cooked
    according to packet
    instructions
2 tbsp plain Greek-style soya
    yogurt alternative

Heat the oil in a large pan, add the onion and cook over a medium
heat for 3–4 minutes until translucent. Add the garlic, ginger and
spices (or curry paste) and cook for 1 minute. Add the cauliflower
and continue cooking for a further 2–3 minutes.

Stir in the tomatoes, beans, apricots and water. Bring to the boil,
then reduce the heat and simmer for 10 minutes until the cauliflower
is tender.

Add the spinach, turn off the heat and leave for 2–3 minutes for the
spinach to wilt down. Stir in the fresh coriander and season to taste.
To serve, scatter over the almonds and serve with basmati rice and
plain yogurt.

NUTRITION per serving	407 cals | 21 g protein | 16 g fat (2 g saturates) | 38 g carbs (20 g total sugars) | 16 g fibre
	Including 50 g (dry weight) basmati rice:
	587 cals | 25 g protein | 16 g fat (2 g saturates) | 77 g carbs (20 g total sugars)• 16 g fibre

PART 2 ● RECIPES

Chickpea masala with spinach

· · · · · · · · · · · ·

Chickpeas make a nutritious base for this curry. They are brilliant sources of protein and carbohydrate, making this a great pre- or post-workout meal. Also, they are rich in fibre, which feeds the beneficial bacteria that live in your gut. Having good gut health is linked to less illness and better sporting performance. I often vary this recipe by substituting different vegetables such as butternut squash, aubergine or sweet potatoes.

SERVES 2

1 tbsp light olive or rapeseed oil
1 onion, sliced
1 tsp cumin seeds
1–2 garlic cloves, crushed
2-cm piece fresh root ginger,
    peeled and grated
1 fresh green chilli, deseeded
    and sliced, or to taste
1 tsp garam masala
1 tsp ground turmeric
1 tsp ground coriander
¼–½ tsp chilli powder (optional)
200 g canned chopped tomatoes
400 g can chickpeas, drained
    and rinsed
Splash of water
100 g baby spinach
Salt and freshly ground black
    pepper, to taste

TO SERVE

A small handful of fresh coriander,
    chopped
Greek-style plain soya yogurt
    alternative and 100 g basmati
    rice, cooked according to
    packet instructions

Heat the oil in a heavy-based saucepan and fry the onion and cumin seeds over a medium heat for 2–3 minutes until softened. Stir in the garlic, ginger and fresh chilli and fry for a few seconds, then add the garam masala, turmeric, ground coriander and chilli powder (if using) and fry for a further minute

If you have time, purée the canned tomatoes with a hand blender (for a smoother sauce although this isn't essential). Add the tomatoes with the chickpeas and a splash of water to the onion mixture and mix well. Bring to the boil, then reduce the heat, cover and simmer for 15 minutes until the sauce has thickened. Season with salt and pepper to taste.

Turn off the heat, stir in the spinach and let it wilt down in the heat of the pan.

Serve garnished with fresh coriander and with the yogurt alternative and basmati rice.

| NUTRITION per serving | 270 cals | 12 g protein | 10 g fat (1 g saturates) | 29 g carbs (9 g total sugars) | 10 g fibre |

Including 1 tbsp Greek-style plain soya yogurt alternative and 50 g (dry weight) basmati rice:
484 cals | **20** g protein | **12** g fat (**2** g saturates) | **70** g carbs (**10** g total sugars) | **11** g fibre

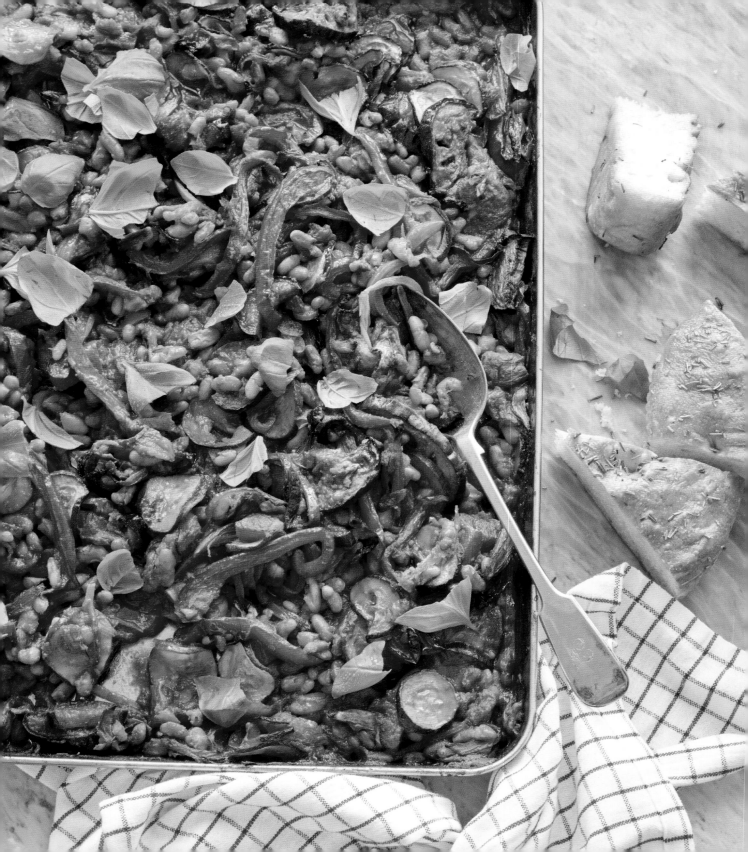

Oven-roasted ratatouille with flageolet beans

....

This is my go-to midweek dish when courgettes are plentiful and in season.
It could not be easier to make – you simply add all the ingredients to a roasting tin and let
the oven do the work. It is packed with beta-carotene, vitamin C, folate and fibre. I have used
flageolet beans (small, immature kidney beans, widely available from supermarkets) in this dish
to boost the protein content but you can easily substitute with chickpeas or any other type of
canned beans. You can also substitute fresh tomatoes for canned when in season and
add a pinch of dried chilli flakes if you like heat.

SERVES 4

1 red onion, thinly sliced
2 red peppers, deseeded and
    sliced
2 large courgettes, thinly sliced
1 large aubergine, sliced into
    half-moons
2 x 400 g cans flageolet beans,
    drained and rinsed
2 garlic cloves, crushed
2 tablespoons extra virgin
    olive oil
1 tbsp balsamic vinegar
2 x 400 g cans chopped
    tomatoes
A handful of basil leaves, torn
Salt and freshly ground black
    pepper, to taste

TO SERVE

Focaccia bread or couscous

Preheat the oven to 200°C/fan 180°C/gas mark 6.

Place the onion, peppers, courgettes, aubergine, flageolet beans and
garlic in a large roasting tin. Season generously with salt and freshly
ground black pepper. Add the olive oil and balsamic vinegar and toss
so that the vegetables are well-coated in the oil. Tip in the tomatoes
and spread out evenly to cover the vegetables.

Transfer to the oven and roast for about 30 minutes. Stir and return
to the oven for a further 30 minutes. Scatter over the basil leaves,
serve hot or cold with wedges of focaccia bread or couscous.

NUTRITION per serving	269 cals | 13 g protein | 7 g fat (1 g saturates) | 33 g carbs (18 g total sugars) | 13 g fibre
	Including 75 g focaccia bread:
	464 cals | 20 g protein | 11 g fat (2 g saturates) | 65 g carbs (20 g total sugars) | 15 g fibre

Pad thai with crispy tofu

· · · · · · · · · · · · · ·

Perfect for fuelling your workout, this nutritious combination of noodles,
tofu and colourful vegetables provides plenty of carbohydrate and protein. It also
gives you your entire daily requirement for vitamin C. I have used pre-marinated tofu
in this recipe as it has a lower moisture and higher protein content than other types
of tofu. If you cannot find it, simply use plain tofu and marinate for a minimum
of 15 minutes before cooking (*see* recipe notes, below).

SERVES 2

150 g rice noodles
2 tbsp sesame or rapeseed oil
160 g marinated tofu, drained
    and cut into 2-cm cubes*
4 spring onions, sliced
1 garlic clove, finely chopped
2-cm piece fresh root ginger,
    grated
½ red chilli, deseeded and sliced,
    or to taste
1 red pepper, deseeded and sliced
2 large handfuls (about 100 g)
    beansprouts
100 g pak choi (Chinese cabbage),
    sliced
1 tbsp tamari (Japanese soy
    sauce) or soy sauce
1 tbsp sweet chilli sauce
Juice of ½ lime

TO SERVE

50 g salted peanuts, crushed
A handful of fresh coriander,
    chopped
Lime, cut into wedges

Cook the noodles according to the pack instructions. Drain and set aside.

Heat half the oil in a wok or large non-stick pan over high heat and fry the tofu cubes for about 2 minutes on each side, until golden all over. Set aside.

Heat the remaining oil over a high heat and fry the spring onions, garlic, ginger, chilli and red pepper for 2–3 minutes. Add the beansprouts and pak choi and continue cooking for 2 minutes. Stir in the cooked noodles, tamari or soy sauce and sweet chilli sauce; cook for 2 minutes more, tossing the noodles until mixed well. Mix in the tofu and lime juice and heat through.

Divide among 2 bowls and scatter over the peanuts, lime wedges and coriander to serve.

* To make your own marinated tofu, mix together 2 tablespoons tamari (Japanese soy sauce) or soy sauce, 1 tablespoon lemon juice or apple cider vinegar, 1 teaspoon grated ginger, 1 teaspoon maple syrup, 1 teaspoon garlic granules and 4 tablespoons water. Spoon the marinade over diced tofu and leave in the fridge for at least 15 minutes, turning occasionally. Remove the tofu from the marinade before using.

NUTRITION per serving | **455** cals | **21** g protein | **19** g fat (**3** g saturates) | **48** g carbs (**9** g total sugars) | **6** g fibre

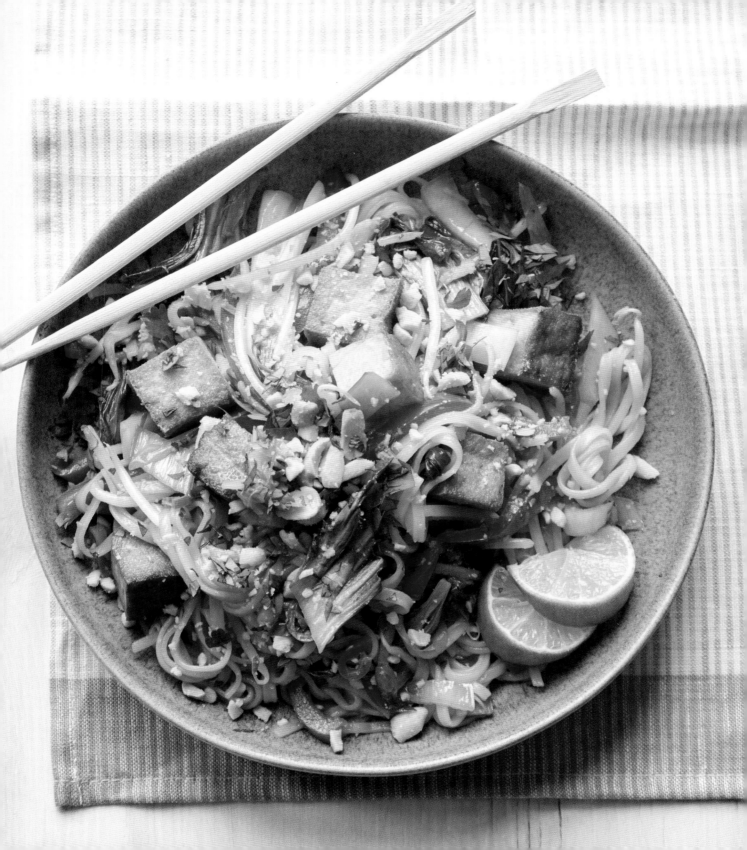

Courgette, edamame and asparagus pasta

. . . .

This tasty pasta dish is ideal before or after an endurance workout or competition.
It is high in carbohydrate and protein, and provides plenty of vitamins C and E, iron and
beta-carotene. The magic is in the sauce. As the pasta cooks, it releases starch, which turns
the courgettes into a tasty, rich sauce. You can substitute frozen peas for the edamame
beans and use any other vegetables you have to hand.

SERVES 2

1 tbsp extra virgin or light olive
    oil, plus extra to serve
2 courgettes, thinly sliced
1 garlic clove, crushed
225 ml vegetable stock
150 ml plant milk alternative
    (any type)
150 g linguine (or any other pasta)
100 g frozen edamame beans
100 g asparagus, cut into 5-cm
    lengths
50 g rocket
A small bunch of parsley, chopped
A few mint leaves, chopped
Juice of ½ lemon
Salt and freshly ground black
    pepper, to taste

TO SERVE

25 g hazelnuts, toasted (p. 57)
Drizzle of olive oil

Heat the oil in a large pan over a low to medium heat. Add the
courgettes and cook gently for 5 minutes until they start to soften.
Add the garlic and continue cooking for 1 minute.

Pour in the stock and the milk, bring to the boil, then add the pasta.
Reduce the heat, cover with a lid and simmer for 10 minutes, or until
the pasta is firm to the bite. Add the edamame beans and asparagus
and cook for a further 3 minutes.

Stir through the rocket, parsley and mint, then season with salt,
freshly ground black pepper and a generous squeeze of lemon juice.

Divide between two bowls, scatter over the toasted hazelnuts and
finish with a drizzle of olive oil.

NUTRITION per serving | **532** cals | **25** g protein | **17** g fat (**2** g saturates) | **65** g carbs (**8** g total sugars) | **11** g fibre

Rainbow stir-fry

. . . .

This colourful stir-fry is super-quick and full of fibre, vitamin C and phytonutrients that promote health and aid muscle adaptation. It provides plenty of protein from four different sources – edamame beans, noodles, cashew nuts and sesame seeds – which makes this dish ideal for post-exercise recovery. It also supplies your daily requirement for vitamins C and E. You can use any other vegetables you have to hand, such as mushrooms, green beans, asparagus, spring onions, green cabbage and bamboo shoots.

SERVES 2

150 g wholewheat noodles
   (egg-free)
1 tbsp light olive or rapeseed oil
½ red onion, sliced
2 garlic cloves, crushed
2-cm piece fresh root ginger,
   finely grated
1 red pepper, thinly sliced
100 g tenderstem broccoli
   (or broccoli florets)
75 g baby sweetcorn
50 g mangetout
100 g frozen edamame beans
1–2 tbsp tamari (Japanese
   soy sauce)
2 tbsp water
Juice of 1 lime

TO SERVE

25 g cashew nuts, toasted (p. 57)
1 tbsp sesame seeds

Cook the noodles in a saucepan according to the instructions on the packet; drain.

Heat the oil in a wok over a high heat until it is hot, add the onion, garlic, ginger and red pepper; stir-fry for 2 minutes. Add the broccoli, sweetcorn and mangetout and stir-fry for 1 minute. Add the edamame and continue stir-frying for 1 minute.

Add the tamari, water and lime juice; stir, then tip in the drained noodles. Continue stir-frying for a further 2 minutes. Remove from the heat and serve in bowls sprinkled with cashew nuts and sesame seeds.

NUTRITION per serving | **596** cals | **26** g protein | **22** g fat (**3** g saturates) | **66** g carbs (**8** g total sugars) | **17** g fibre

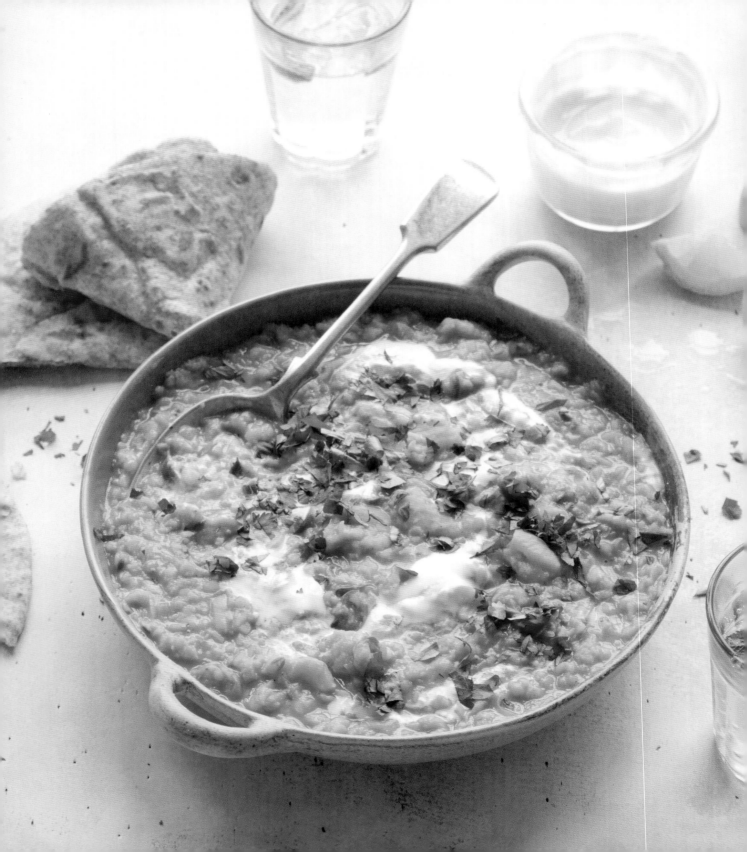

Red lentil dal

....

*Dal – **essentially cooked lentils** – is warming, full of flavour and a brilliant way of getting lots of fibre that's so important for nurturing the gut microbiota, along with plenty of protein and iron. One serving provides more than one third of a female athlete's daily requirement for iron. This recipe is incredibly versatile and can be varied every time by adding different vegetables. I like to add spinach just before serving as it provides a beautiful colour contrast – as well as vitamin C and folate – but you can also add diced butternut squash, cauliflower, sliced carrots, potatoes, or whatever you have available when you add the red lentils to the pan. Cashews add extra protein, but you can substitute toasted almonds or pecans.*

SERVES 4

1 tbsp light olive or rapeseed oil
1 onion, finely chopped
1 tsp cumin seeds
2 garlic cloves, crushed
5-cm piece fresh root ginger, peeled and grated
1 red chilli, deseeded and finely sliced, or to taste
1 tsp turmeric
1 tsp garam masala
200 g red lentils
500 ml hot water
400 ml can light coconut milk
6 dried apricots, roughly chopped
100 g baby spinach
50 g cashew nuts
Juice of ½ lemon
A small bunch of fresh coriander, chopped
Salt and freshly ground black pepper, to taste

TO SERVE

200 g basmati rice or 4 chapatis, plain soya yogurt alternative (optional)

Heat the oil in a heavy-based pan over a medium heat. Add the onion and fry for 4–5 minutes until translucent. Stir in the cumin seeds, garlic, ginger, chilli, turmeric and garam masala. Continue cooking for 1 further minute, stirring continuously.

Add the lentils, hot water, coconut milk and apricots; bring to the boil, cover and reduce to a simmer. Cook for about 20 minutes, stirring occasionally. Turn off the heat and stir in the spinach (it will wilt down and cook in the heat of the pan).

Stir in the cashew nuts and lemon juice and season with salt and freshly ground black pepper. Finally, stir in the fresh coriander. Serve with a swirl of plain yogurt alternative, basmati rice or chapatis.

NUTRITION per serving	393 cals	17 g protein	17 g fat (8 g saturates)	39 g carbs (10 g total sugars)	6 g fibre
	Including 50 g (dry weight) basmati rice:				
	573 cals	21 g protein	18 g fat (8 g saturates)	79 g carbs (10 g total sugars)	7 g fibre
	Including 1 chapati:				
	568 cals	22 g protein	23 g fat (11 g saturates)	64 g carbs (13 g total sugars)	10 g fibre

Satay noodles

....

Full of flavour and crunch, this easy stir-fry recipe is my go-to meal before any endurance workout. It combines noodles with tofu, colourful vegetables and a tasty satay sauce, so provides a perfect balance of carbohydrate, protein and healthy fats that will keep you fuelled during exercise. It also supplies plenty of fibre, vitamin C and calcium. You can swap the tofu for edamame beans or peas, or add different vegetables such as broccoli, mushrooms, courgettes or thinly sliced cabbage.

SERVES 4

2 tbsp light olive or rapeseed oil
200 g firm tofu, drained and cut into 2-cm cubes
6 spring onions, sliced on the diagonal
1-cm piece fresh root ginger, peeled and finely grated
2 garlic cloves, crushed
2 carrots, cut into thin batons
2 peppers (ideally, different colours), deseeded and thinly sliced
200 g sugar snap peas
200 g wholewheat noodles (egg-free)

FOR THE SATAY SAUCE

75 g peanut butter
A pinch of chilli flakes
2 tbsp tamari (Japanese soy sauce) or soy sauce
1 tbsp maple syrup
Juice of 1 lime
4 tbsp water

TO SERVE

A handful of fresh coriander, chopped
50 g roughly chopped peanuts

Cook the noodles in a large saucepan of boiling water according to the directions on the packet. Drain and set aside.

Heat 1 tablespoon of the oil in a wok over high heat and fry the tofu cubes for about 2 minutes on each side until golden all over. Set aside.

Use a fork to whisk all the satay sauce ingredients together in a bowl, adding an extra splash of water if needed.

Heat the remaining oil over a high heat and add the spring onions, ginger, garlic, carrots, peppers and sugar snap peas. Stir-fry for 2–3 minutes until they are slightly charred but still firm.

Add the noodles to the wok. Pour in the sauce and tofu and cook for another 1–2 minutes, tossing the noodles until mixed well. Serve sprinkled with coriander and peanuts.

NUTRITION per serving | **563** cals | **25** g protein | **27** g fat (**5** g saturates) | **49** g carbs (**12** g total sugars) | **12** g fibre

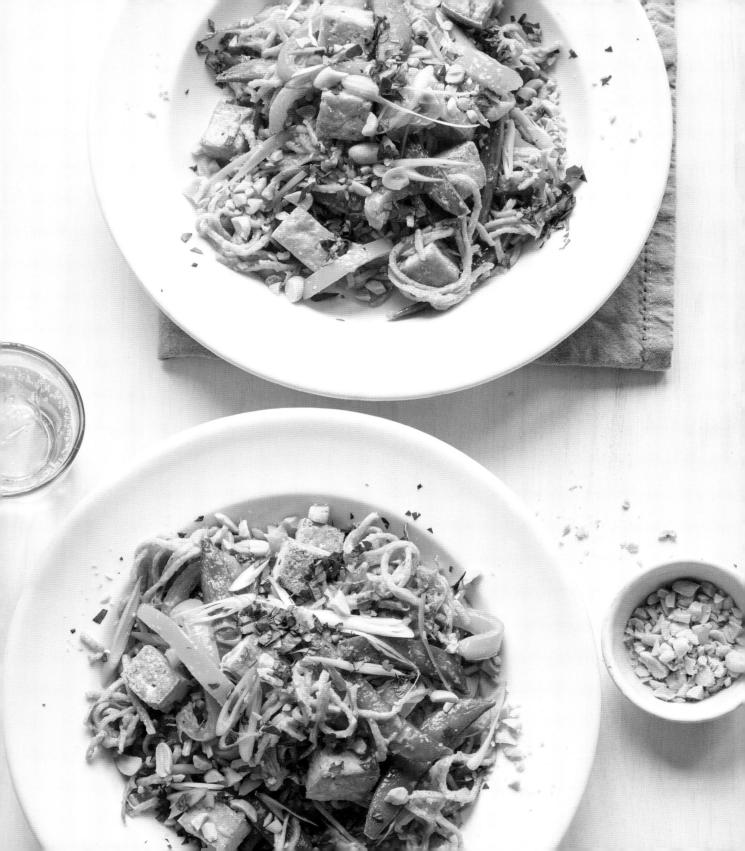

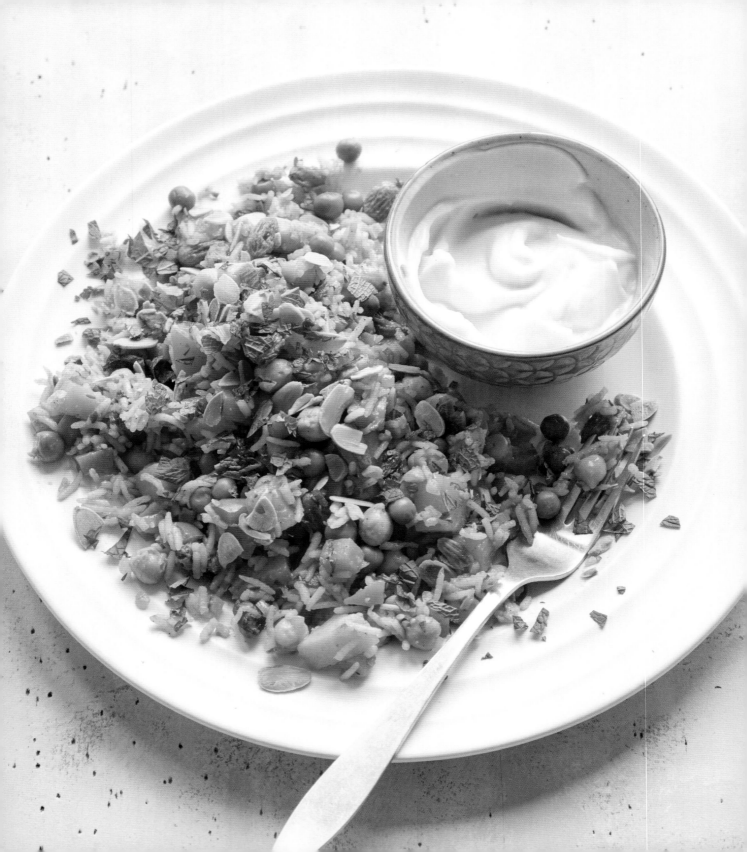

Spiced chickpea pilaff with almonds and coconut yogurt

············

This tasty combination of rice, chickpeas and almonds is an ideal pre-exercise meal that will sustain you through your workout. Chickpeas are nutritional powerhouses, packed with carbohydrate, protein, fibre, B vitamins, iron, zinc and magnesium. They are the perfect nutritional complement to rice, balancing out the shortfall of essential amino acids and raising the overall quality of protein. Carrots and butternut squash are both rich in beta-carotene, while green peppers and peas are loaded with vitamin C. Almonds add additional protein, healthy fats, calcium and vitamin E. Substitute pecans or cashews if you prefer. If you don't have all the individual spices, then use 2 tablespoons of mild curry paste instead.

SERVES 2

1 tbsp light olive or rapeseed oil

1 small onion, finely chopped

½ green or red pepper, deseeded and chopped

1 garlic clove, crushed

2-cm piece fresh root ginger, grated

1 tsp cumin seeds

1 tsp each: ground cumin, ground coriander and garam masala

½ tsp turmeric

¼ tsp dried chilli flakes

1 large carrot, diced

¼ butternut squash (approximately 250 g), peeled and cut into 1-cm cubes

100 g basmati rice

300 ml hot vegetable stock or water

400 g can chickpeas, drained and rinsed

25 g sultanas

75 g frozen peas

TO SERVE

25 g almonds, toasted and crushed (p. 57)

Small handful finely chopped mint

2 tbsp coconut yogurt alternative

Heat the oil in a large non-stick pan and fry the onion and green pepper over a gentle heat for 5 minutes. Add the garlic, ginger, cumin seeds and the remaining spices; continue cooking for 1 minute.

Add the vegetables and rice. Mix together until coated in the spices, then add the vegetable stock or water, chickpeas and sultanas. Stir well, bring to the boil, then reduce the heat, cover and simmer for about 10–12 minutes until most of the liquid has been absorbed and the rice and vegetables are tender. Make sure the mixture does not boil dry; add extra water, if necessary. Add the peas for the last 3 minutes of cooking.

Serve topped with the almonds and chopped mint, and a spoonful of coconut yogurt alternative.

| NUTRITION per serving | **652** cals | **23** g protein | **18** g fat (**2** g saturates) | **91** g carbs (**25** g total sugars) | **18** g fibre |

Sri Lankan sambar curry

....

This vegan Sri Lankan curry has a wonderfully rich and fragrant flavour, thanks to the garlic, ginger, chilli, and curry spices. The coconut milk works as a stock, absorbing all the delicious spicy flavours to create a wonderful sauce for the vegetables. Sweet potatoes are rich in carbohydrate and beta-carotene, which has powerful antioxidant properties. I have added lentils to help thicken the sauce as well as providing protein, fibre and iron. Broccoli is a rich source of vitamin C, folate and iron, but you can substitute spinach if you prefer.

PART 2 • RECIPES

SERVES 4

2 medium sweet potatoes,
   scrubbed and cut into cubes
¼ butternut squash
   (approximately 250 g), peeled
   and cut into 1-cm cubes
2 tbsp light olive or rapeseed oil
1 red onion, finely chopped
2–3 garlic cloves, crushed
5-cm piece fresh root ginger,
   grated
2 red chillies, deseeded and
   sliced, or to taste
½ tsp cumin seeds
½ tsp black mustard seeds
5 cardamom pods, crushed
6–8 curry leaves (optional)
1 tsp turmeric
1 tsp ground coriander
400 ml can light coconut milk
250 ml hot water
125 g red lentils
200 g tenderstem broccoli
Juice of 1 lime
A handful of fresh coriander,
   chopped
Salt

TO SERVE

200 g basmati rice (cooked
   according to packet
   instructions)
4 tbsp Greek-style plain soya
   yogurt alternative

Preheat the oven to 200°C/fan 180°C/gas mark 6. Place the prepared sweet potatoes and butternut squash on a baking tray. Sprinkle over a little salt, add 1 tablespoon of the oil and toss so all vegetables are well-coated. Roast in the oven for about 25 minutes until soft.

Meanwhile, heat the remaining 1 tablespoon oil in a large pan over a low to medium heat. Add the onion and fry gently for 5 minutes until translucent. Add the garlic, ginger, chillies, cumin and mustard seeds. Continue cooking for 1 minute, stirring continuously, before adding the cardamom pods, curry leaves, turmeric and ground coriander; cook for another minute. Add the coconut milk, hot water and lentils. Bring to the boil, then reduce the heat and simmer for 15 minutes. Add the broccoli and cook for another 5 minutes.

Add the roasted vegetables. Stir in the lime juice and coriander (reserve a little to serve) and season with salt to taste. Serve with cooked basmati rice and yogurt alternative, and scatter over the remaining coriander.

NUTRITION per serving	356 cals | 12 g protein | 14 g fat (7 g saturates) | 41 g carbs (11 g total sugars) | 8 g fibre
	Including 50 g (dry weight) basmati rice and 1 tablespoon yogurt alternative: 569 cals | 20 g protein | 16 g fat (8 g saturates) | 82 g carbs (12 g total sugars) | 10 g fibre

Thai green curry with crispy tofu balls

· · · · · · · · · · · ·

These crispy tofu balls made with tofu and cashews are easy to make and an excellent source of protein and calcium. In this recipe, I have combined them with a delicious Thai green curry sauce made in a blender to save time. Pak choi (Chinese cabbage) provides plenty of vitamin C and folate. You can also add different vegetables, such as broccoli, sliced green cabbage or mushrooms.

SERVES 2

40 g cashew nuts
25 g fresh breadcrumbs
200 g firm tofu
4 spring onions, sliced
1 tbsp light olive or rapeseed oil
1 courgette, sliced
100 g baby corn
100 g mangetout
1 head pak choi (Chinese cabbage), cut into large pieces
Salt and freshly ground black pepper, to taste

FOR THE CURRY SAUCE

1 spring onion, sliced
2-cm piece fresh root ginger, roughly chopped
Juice of ½ lime
A handful of coriander, roughly chopped (reserve a little to garnish)
2 garlic cloves, crushed
1 tsp sugar
2 tsp tamari (Japanese soy sauce) or soy sauce
½ red or green chilli, deseeded, to taste
200 ml canned coconut milk
50 ml vegetable stock or water

TO SERVE

1 lime, cut into wedges
A handful of fresh coriander, chopped
Cooked noodles (optional)

Preheat the oven to 180°C/fan 160°C/gas mark 4. Place the cashews on a baking tray and bake in the oven for 7–9 minutes until lightly toasted. When they are ready, remove from the oven and allow to cool a little.

Tip half the cashews into the bowl of a food processor (reserve the rest for the garnish) and pulse a few times to break up. Add the breadcrumbs, tofu and the spring onions; blend until the ingredients begin to clump together. Shape into about 20 small balls.

Heat the oil in the frying pan and fry the tofu balls, shaking the pan frequently for about 5 minutes until lightly browned. Tip out onto a plate.

To make the curry sauce, place the spring onion, ginger, lime juice, coriander, garlic, sugar, tamari or soy sauce, chilli, coconut milk and vegetable stock or water in the bowl of a blender. Blend until smooth. Transfer the sauce to a large pan and bring to the boil.

Add the courgette, baby corn and mangetout. Bring to the boil, reduce the heat, cover and simmer for 3–4 minutes, then add the pak choi. Continue cooking for 1 minute. Taste and season with salt and pepper.

Divide the curry into bowls and top with the remaining cashews and coriander. Serve with lime wedges and the tofu balls on the side (don't mix into the curry otherwise they will break up) and cooked noodles, if liked.

NUTRITION per serving | **563** cals | **25** g protein | **40** g fat (**19** g saturates) | **22** g carbs (**11** g total sugars) | **8** g fibre

Three-bean chilli with cashew cream

. . . .

This delicious, spicy chilli has everything you need to help you hit your PBs. Beans contain plenty of protein and carbohydrates to boost energy, tomatoes provide lycopene for heart health, and the beta-carotene in carrots supports healthy immunity and good eye health. Plus, it's full of fibre that feeds the beneficial microbes in your gut, lowers cancer risk and supports healthy immunity. Any leftovers will keep in the fridge for up to three days or you can freeze for up to three months.

SERVES 4

1 tbsp light olive or rapeseed oil
1 small onion, finely chopped
1–2 garlic cloves, crushed
½–1 tsp chilli powder, or to taste
1 tbsp sweet paprika
1 tsp dried oregano
1 tsp ground cumin
2 celery sticks, finely sliced
2 carrots, diced
100 g mushrooms, chopped
2 x 400 g cans chopped
    tomatoes
2 tbsp tomato purée
300 ml vegetable stock
400 g can red kidney beans,
    drained and rinsed
400 g can black beans, drained
    and rinsed
400 g can chickpeas, drained
    and rinsed
Salt and freshly ground pepper,
    to taste

TO SERVE

A handful of fresh parsley,
    chopped
4 tbsp (½ quantity) Cashew
    Cream (p. 178)
200 g basmati rice (cooked
    according to packet
    instructions)

Heat the oil in a large non-stick pan over a medium heat. Add the onion and fry for 3–4 minutes until translucent. Add the garlic, chilli powder, paprika, oregano and cumin and cook for a further 1 minute. Add the celery, carrots and mushrooms and continue cooking for 1–2 minutes. Tip in the tomatoes, tomato purée, vegetable stock, beans and chickpeas, stir well and bring to the boil. Reduce the heat and simmer for around 20 minutes until the vegetables are tender and the flavours have blended together.

Season with salt and freshly ground pepper. Sprinkle with chopped parsley and serve with a spoonful of Cashew Cream and basmati rice.

NUTRITION per serving	413 cals	21 g protein	13 g fat (2 g saturates)	45 g carbs (14 g total sugars)	18 g fibre
	Including 50 g (dry weight) basmati rice:				
	593 cals	25 g protein	13 g fat (2 g saturates)	85 g carbs (14 g total sugars)	18 g fibre

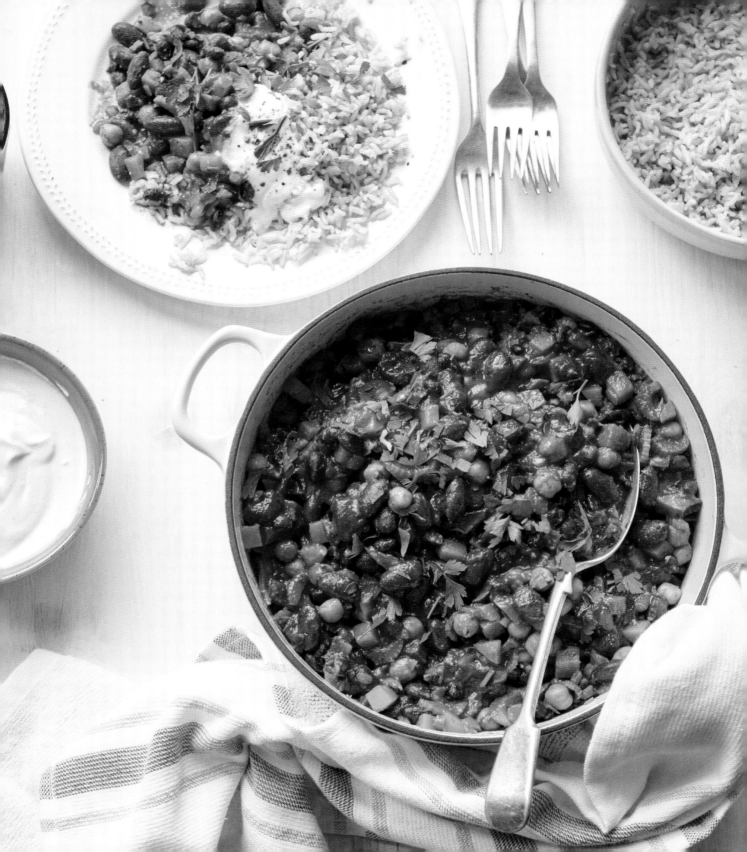

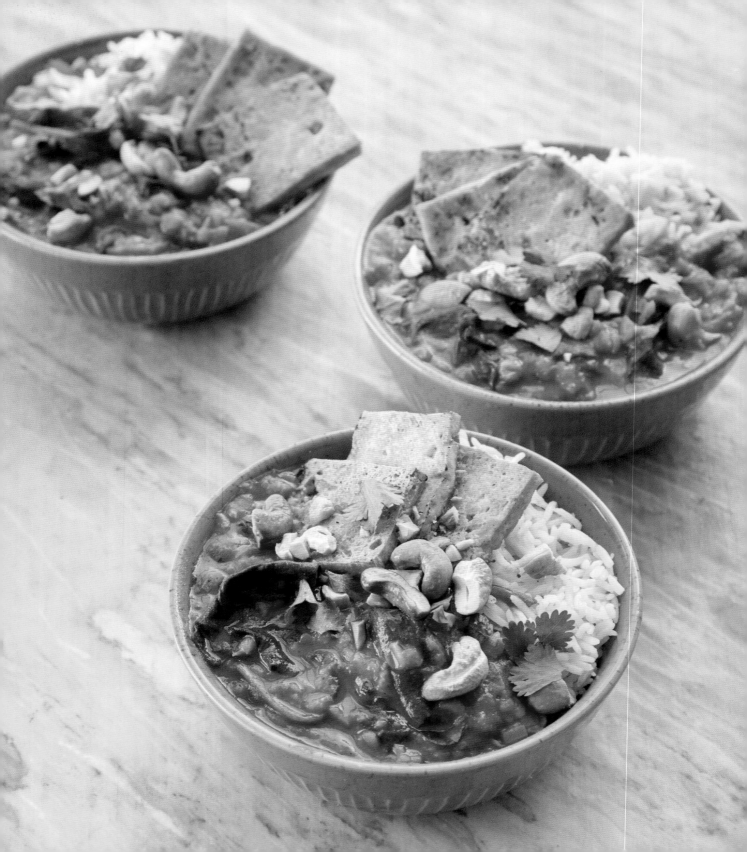

Tomato and coconut dal with crispy tofu and cashews

·············

This simple dal includes three different protein sources – lentils, tofu and cashews – which provide an excellent balance of essential amino acids, making this an ideal dish for muscle growth and recovery. One serving of this dal also provides one third of a female's daily requirement for iron, a mineral needed for making haemoglobin, the oxygen-carrying protein in red blood cells, and preventing iron-deficiency anaemia. Uptake by the body is enhanced by vitamin C from the canned tomatoes and spinach.

SERVES 4

3 tbsp light olive or rapeseed oil
1 large onion, finely diced
2 garlic cloves, crushed
2-cm piece fresh root ginger, peeled and grated
1 small red chilli, deseeded and finely chopped, or to taste
1 tbsp garam masala
200 g red lentils, rinsed
300 ml hot water
1–2 tsp vegetable bouillon powder
400 g can tomatoes
400 ml can light coconut milk
100 g baby spinach
A large handful of fresh coriander, chopped, plus extra to garnish
200 g firm tofu, sliced

TO SERVE

50 g cashews, toasted (p. 57)
200 g basmati rice (cooked according to packet instructions)

Heat 2 tablespoons of the oil in a large saucepan over a medium-low heat, add the onion and fry for 4–5 minutes until translucent. Add the garlic, ginger, chilli and garam masala; continue cooking for a further minute, stirring continuously.

Add the lentils, hot water, bouillon powder and tomatoes. Bring to the boil. Cover and simmer for about 20 minutes, stirring frequently so the lentils don't stick to the bottom of the pan (add more water if needed). Add the coconut milk, turn off the heat and stir in the spinach. It will wilt down and cook in the heat of the pan. Finally, stir in the fresh coriander.

Heat the remaining 1 tablespoon olive oil and fry the tofu slices for 5–6 minutes until browned on both sides. Serve on top of the dal and scatter over the cashews and extra coriander.

NUTRITION per serving	**498** cals | **24** g protein | **27** g fat (**9** g saturates) | **38** g carbs (**9** g total sugars) | **7** g fibre
	Including 50 g (dry weight) basmati rice: **678** cals | **28** g protein | **27** g fat (**10** g saturates) | **78** g carbs (**9** g total sugars) | **7** g fibre

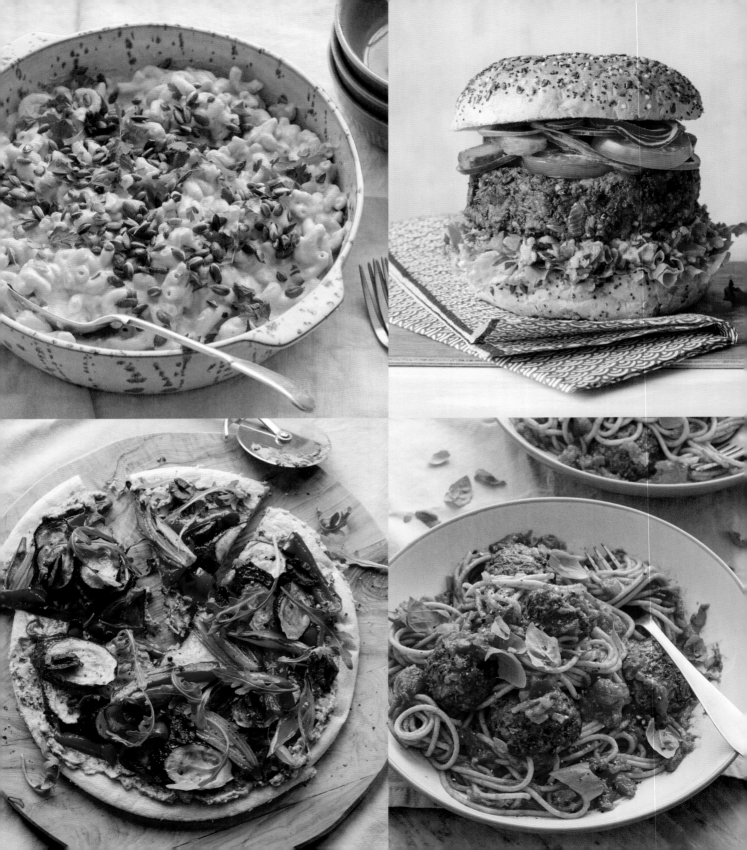

Weekend dinners

Clockwise from top left: Butternut macaroni cheese; Black bean
burgers with guacamole; Lentil and mushroom no-meatballs in
tomato sauce; Chickpea pizza with basil pesto and olives.

Black bean burgers with guacamole

....

'So, what do you eat at a BBQ then?' is a question I get asked at every BBQ party. In reply, I point them to this scrumptious recipe, which is guaranteed to satisfy the most sceptical non-vegan. Made with black beans and walnuts, these easy burgers are full of amazing flavour and a brilliant source of plant protein, fibre, folate, magnesium and iron. Serve on a bun with all the trimmings or with grilled slices of courgettes and aubergines, and toasted flatbread.

MAKES 4 LARGE OR 8 SMALL BURGERS

50 g wholegrain bread
75 g walnuts
2 tbsp extra virgin olive oil
2 large shallots or ½ red onion, finely chopped
1 small aubergine, cut into 1-cm dice
1 small carrot, grated
1 garlic clove, crushed
400 g can black beans, drained and rinsed
1 tsp smoked paprika
1 tsp ground cumin
½ tsp ground cinnamon
¼ tsp cayenne, or to taste
1 tbsp lemon juice
3 tbsp finely chopped coriander
Seeded wholemeal buns
Salt and freshly ground black pepper, to taste

FOR THE GUACAMOLE

1 large ripe avocado
1 tbsp lemon or lime juice
¼ red onion, finely chopped
½ garlic clove, crushed
1 tomato, skinned* and chopped
1 tbsp fresh coriander, finely chopped

To make the burgers, tear the bread into large pieces, add to the bowl of a food processor and process until you have breadcrumbs. Transfer to a mixing bowl and set aside. Add the walnuts to the food processor, pulse until crumbly (but not too fine), then tip into the mixing bowl with the breadcrumbs.

Heat 1 tablespoon of the oil in a large frying pan over a high heat and fry the shallots or red onion, aubergine and grated carrot for 5 minutes, stirring frequently. Add the garlic and continue cooking for 1 further minute.

Tip the mixture into the bowl of the food processor with the beans, spices, lemon juice, salt and freshly ground black pepper; process for about 30 seconds or until you have a coarse purée. It should not be totally smooth – you still want some whole beans in there for texture. Transfer to the bowl with the breadcrumbs and walnuts and mix in the coriander.

Use a large spoon to scoop out 4 or 8 patties and flatten them into round shapes. Transfer to a large plate and place in the fridge for 30 minutes to firm up.

Brush the patties with the remaining 1 tablespoon oil and grill on a BBQ or fry in a large, non-stick frying pan over a medium heat for 5 minutes on each side until golden. Alternatively bake in a preheated oven at 190°C/fan 170°C/gas mark 5 for 25 minutes.

For the guacamole, halve the avocado, remove the stone and scoop out the flesh into a bowl. Mash with the lemon or lime juice. Stir through the onion, garlic, tomato, coriander and seasoning.

Serve the burgers on wholemeal seeded buns with a spoonful of guacamole and tomatoes, red onion, lettuce and pickles, if you like.

*To skin the tomato, make a cross in the skin at the base, plunge into a bowl of just boiled water for 30–60 seconds. Remove the tomato from the water and peel with a sharp knife. The skin should come away easily.

NUTRITION per large burger	310 cals	10 g protein	19 g fat (2 g saturates)	20 g carbs (4 g total sugars)	8 g fibre
	Including 1 wholemeal bun and 1 tablespoon guacamole: 593 cals	20 g protein	33 g fat (5 g saturates)	45 g carbs (7 g total sugars)	16 g fibre

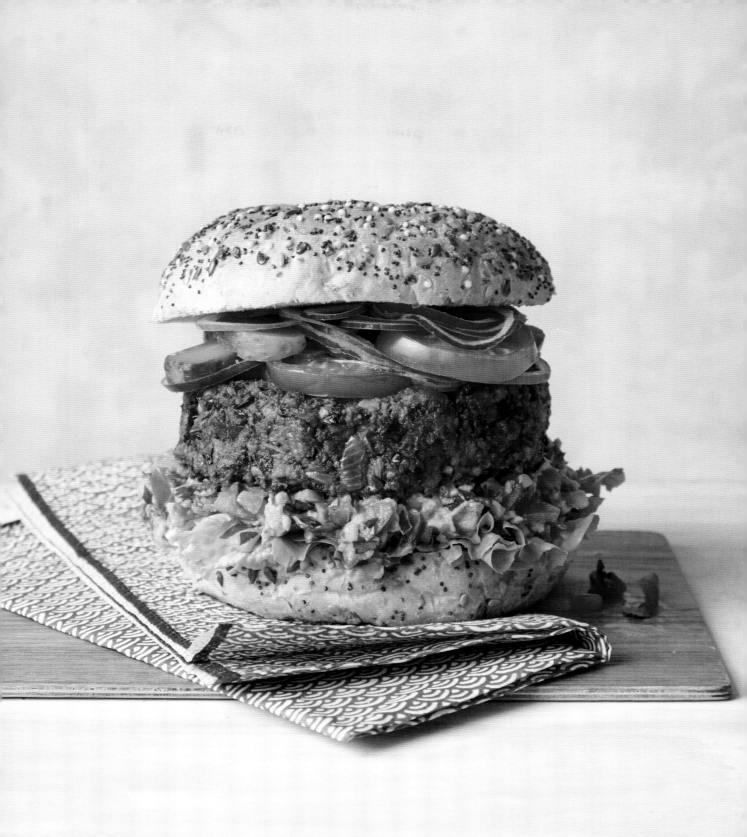

Butternut and walnut galette

· · · · · · · · · · · · · ·

Perfect for Christmas dinner or Sunday lunch, this vegan centrepiece is a great source
of beta-carotene, omega-3s and fibre, and full of delicious flavours. Za'ater, a Middle-Eastern
blend of herbs, sumac and sesame seeds, gives the galette a wonderful aromatic flavour.

SERVES 6

½ butternut squash (approximately
    500 g), peeled, deseeded and cut
    into half-moons, 1-cm thick
4 shallots or 1 small onion, cut into
    wedges
4 tbsp olive oil
1 courgette, sliced
100 g asparagus spears, cut into
    2-cm lengths
1 tsp za'atar (or dried thyme or
    oregano)
40 g walnuts
1 tsp runny honey
Pinch of dried chilli flakes
½ quantity Cashew Cream (p. 178)
A handful of rocket
Salt and freshly ground black pepper,
    to taste

FOR THE PASTRY

40 g walnuts
200 g plain flour, plus extra for
    rolling out
½ tsp salt
100 g dairy-free spread, cut into
    1-cm cubes
4–5 tbsp water

TO SERVE

900 g each roast potatoes and
    Brussels sprouts, if liked

Preheat the oven to 200°C/fan 180°C/gas mark 6.

To make the pastry, blitz the walnuts in a food processor. Add the flour, salt and dairy-free spread; pulse until the mixture resembles fine breadcrumbs. Add 4 tablespoons of the water and pulse until the mixture just comes together to form a dough, adding the remaining water if needed.

Turn the pastry onto a lightly floured surface and knead until it forms a ball. Wrap in cling film and place in the fridge while you make the filling.

Place the butternut squash in a roasting tin with the shallots or onion and season well. Drizzle over 1 tablespoon of the olive oil, toss to coat and season once more. Roast for 20 minutes.

Meanwhile, place the courgette and asparagus spears in another roasting tin, drizzle over 1 tablespoon of the olive oil, sprinkle with za'atar and toss to coat. Roast for 10 minutes.

Remove the butternut squash from the oven, add the walnuts and roast for a further 8 minutes.

Tip half the butternut squash and walnut mixture into a food processor. Add the honey and chilli flakes and blitz on a high speed. While the processor is running, drizzle in the remaining 2 tablespoons olive oil. Check the seasoning and adjust with salt and pepper to taste.

Roll out the pastry to a rough 25-cm circle. Transfer to a baking tray lined with baking paper. Spoon the butternut mixture into the centre of the pastry, leaving a border of about 4 cm around the edge. Arrange the remaining roasted butternut squash, courgettes and asparagus on top of the filling. Fold the pastry border up around the edge of the vegetables. Bake for 30 minutes.

Remove the galette from the oven and dot the top with Cashew Cream. Scatter with rocket and serve with roast potatoes and Brussels sprouts.

NUTRITION per serving	492 cals | 11 g protein | 33 g fat (6 g saturates) | 37 g carbs (7 g total sugars) | 5 g fibre
	Including 150 g each roast potatoes and brussels sprouts:
	824 cals | 20 g protein | 43 g fat (7 g saturates) | 80 g carbs (13 g total sugars) | 18 g fibre

Chickpea kofte kebabs with spiced yogurt

....

These healthy kebabs make a tasty alternative to the traditional takeaway. They are made with chickpeas and tahini, both great sources of protein, fibre, B vitamins, magnesium and iron. Tahini also supplies plenty of calcium, making these kebabs perfect after-match or post-race food. Toasted spices and fresh mint make them light and aromatic. I love serving them in pittas with spiced yogurt (simply dial down the hot sauce if you don't like heat), lots of salad and roasted peppers.

SERVES 4

2 tsp cumin seeds
2 tsp coriander seeds
½ tsp cardamom seeds
400 g can of chickpeas, drained and rinsed
2 garlic cloves
½ red onion, roughly chopped
½ tsp cinnamon
3 tbsp rolled oats
A small handful of mint leaves
60 g tahini
Juice of ½ lemon
3 tbsp olive oil
Salt and freshly ground black pepper, to taste

FOR THE DRESSING

250 g coconut yogurt alternative
1–2 tsp hot chilli sauce (or to taste)
Salt and freshly ground black pepper, to taste

TO SERVE

4 wholemeal pitta breads, mixed salad leaves and roasted red peppers (from a jar)

In a large non-stick frying pan over a medium heat, toast the seeds for 3 minutes then blitz in a blender.

Add the chickpeas, garlic, onion, cinnamon, oats, mint leaves, tahini, lemon juice and a large pinch of salt and pepper.

Pulse until the mixture comes together in clumps but avoid over-processing to a paste. It should stick together well in your hands. If not, add a little water. Divide into 8 and shape into thick sausage-like shapes. Place in the fridge at least 1 hour to firm up.

Heat the olive oil in a large frying pan over a medium heat. Add the kofte and fry for 10–12 minutes, turning every minute or so until golden brown and crispy all over. Alternatively, bake in a preheated oven (180°C/ fan 160°C/ gas mark 4) for 15 minutes until golden.

Meanwhile, make the tahini dressing by mixing the coconut yogurt, hot chilli sauce and a pinch of salt and pepper.

To serve, warm the pitta breads in the oven or a toaster. Fill with salad leaves and roasted red peppers, then top with the koftes and drizzle over the spicy yogurt dressing.

NUTRITION per serving* | **548** cals | **20** g protein | **23** g fat (**4** g saturates) | **60** g carbs (**6** g total sugars) | **13** g fibre

*including 1 pitta, ¼ jar red peppers and a handful of salad leaves

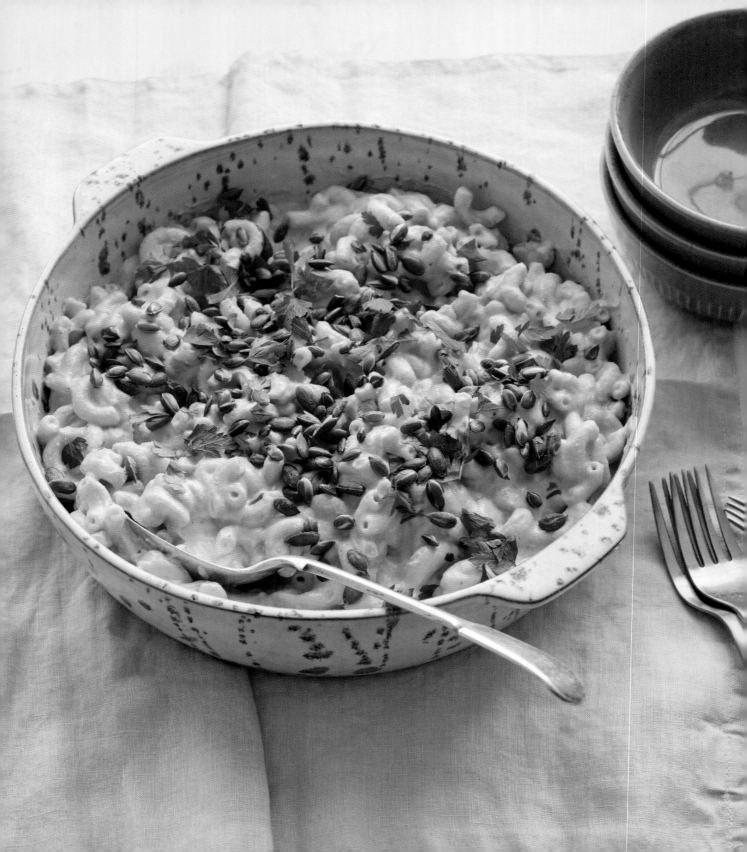

Butternut macaroni cheese

. . . .

I've tried many vegan versions of this classic dish, but none have hit the mark until now. The secret ingredient, it turns out, is butternut squash. It becomes incredibly velvety and beautifully sweet when cooked and, when blended with cashews, makes a perfect vegan substitute for cheese sauce. It also happens to be packed with beta-carotene, a powerful antioxidant that promotes muscle recovery. Cashews are rich in healthy fats, protein and iron, while nutritional yeast is a great source of B vitamins, also adding a lovely cheesy flavour. I have topped this dish with pumpkin seeds for extra omega-3 fats.

SERVES 4

½ butternut squash
(approximately 500 g), peeled
and cut into small pieces
1 small onion, chopped
2 whole garlic cloves
2 tbsp light olive or rapeseed oil
300 g macaroni (or similar pasta
shape)
150 g cashews, soaked overnight
(or in boiling water for 1 hour)
125 ml almond milk alternative
3 tbsp nutritional yeast flakes
Squeeze of lemon juice
Salt and freshly ground black
pepper, to taste

TO SERVE

40 g toasted pumpkin seeds
(p. 57)
A handful of chopped parsley

Preheat the oven to 200°C/fan 180°C/gas mark 6.

Place the butternut squash, onion and garlic in a large roasting tin, toss with the olive oil and roast in oven for about 25 minutes or until soft. Meanwhile, cook the macaroni according to the packet instructions, then drain.

Drain the cashews and tip them into the bowl of a food processor or high-speed blender and process, adding the almond milk slowly until you have a smooth consistency. Add the roasted vegetables and the remaining ingredients (apart from the pasta); continue to process until silky, adding a little more almond milk until completely smooth.

Toss with the hot macaroni and serve topped with toasted pumpkin seeds and chopped parsley.

NUTRITION per serving | **682** cals | **24** g protein | **30** g fat (**5** g saturates) | **75** g carbs (**10** g total sugars) | **10** g fibre

Cashew, apricot and sage nut roast

....

I have made this tasty nut roast every Christmas for the past five years and always get showered with compliments from both vegan and non-vegan guests. It is crammed with nuts and seeds, which are brilliant sources of healthy fats, protein, fibre, vitamin E, B vitamins and iron. Feel free to substitute different nuts, such as walnuts, Brazils or peanuts, if you prefer. You can replace the mushrooms with leeks, celery or aubergine.

SERVES 6

1 tbsp olive oil
1 medium onion, finely chopped
2 garlic cloves, crushed
1 red or yellow pepper, deseeded
    and finely chopped
75 g mushrooms, chopped
1 large carrot, grated
100 g cashew nuts
100 g almonds (whole or flaked)
50 g mixed seeds
125 g wholemeal breadcrumbs
1 tsp yeast extract (e.g. Marmite)
    dissolved in 100 ml hot water
1 tsp soy sauce
50 g dried apricots, finely
    chopped
2 tbsp ground flaxseeds mixed
    with 6 tbsp water
1 tbsp finely chopped fresh sage
    (or rosemary)
1 tbsp chopped fresh parsley

TO SERVE

900 g each roast potatoes,
Brussels sprouts and 180 ml
vegan gravy (3 tsp vegan gravy
granules with 180 ml boiling
water)

Preheat the oven to 180°C/fan 160°C/gas mark 4. Meanwhile, line a 900 g loaf tin with baking paper.

Heat the olive oil over a moderate heat in a non-stick frying pan, then add the onion and fry for 3 minutes until translucent. Add the garlic and cook for a further 30 seconds. Add the red pepper, mushrooms and carrots and continue cooking for 5 minutes.

Place the cashews and almonds in the bowl of a food processor and pulse until they are chopped but not so much that they turn into flour – you want the pieces of nuts to be a bit chunky. In a large bowl, combine the nuts with the cooked vegetables and all the remaining ingredients.

Spoon the mixture into the lined loaf tin, press down well, cover with foil and bake for 30 minutes. Remove the foil and bake for a further 15 minutes, until firm and golden. Leave it to cool in the tin for about 15 minutes before turning out.

Serve with roast potatoes, Brussels sprouts and vegan gravy.

NUTRITION per serving	383 cals	14 g protein	25 g fat (3 g saturates)	21 g carbs (9 g total sugars)	9 g fibre

Including 150 g each roast potatoes and Brussels sprouts, and 2 tablespoons vegan gravy:
723 cals | **23** g protein | **36** g fat (**4** g saturates) | **66** g carbs (**16** g total sugars) | **21** g fibre

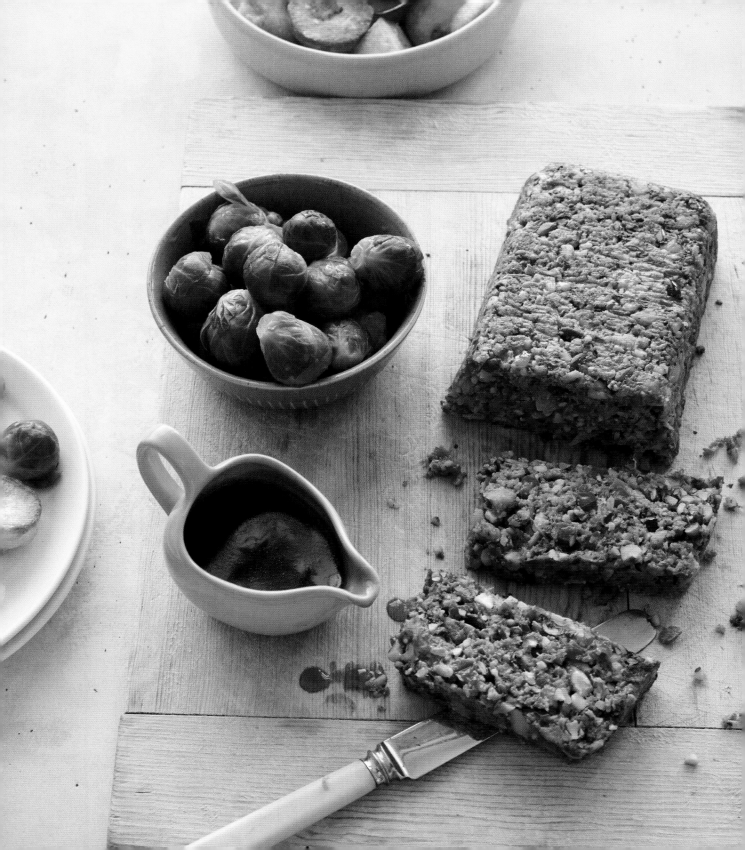

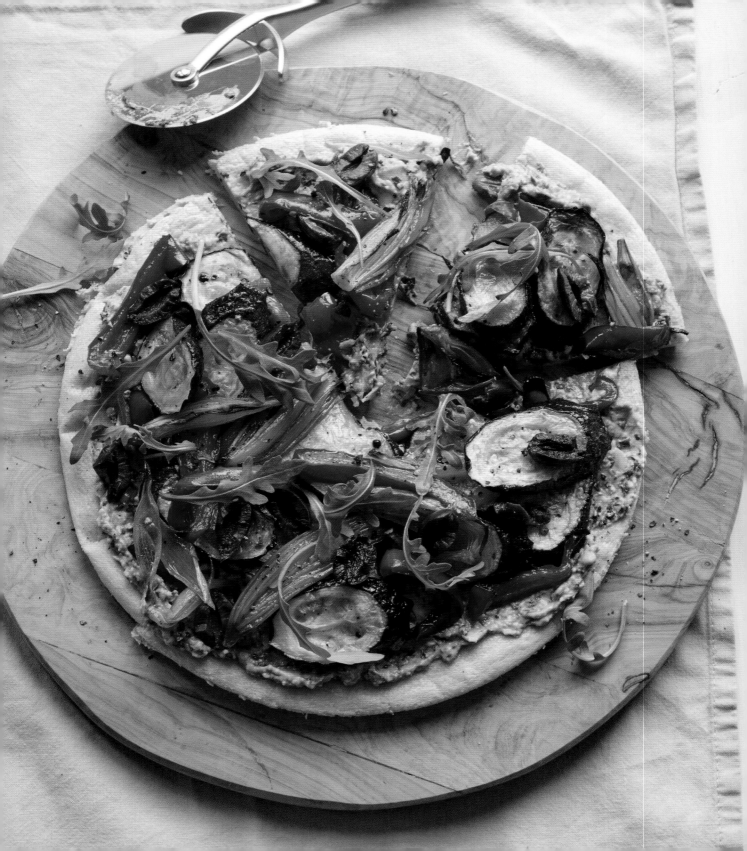

Chickpea pizza with basil pesto and olives

....

I don't always have the time or the patience to make a yeast-based pizza dough so in this recipe I use a chickpea base, which requires no kneading and takes just minutes to make. Chickpea (gram) flour is simply ground chickpeas and is widely available from supermarkets. It is high in protein, fibre and iron, which makes it a nutritious alternative to the wheat flour used for traditional pizzas. You can top with any other vegetables, such as tomatoes, mushrooms or asparagus.

SERVES 2

2 courgettes, sliced diagonally
1 red or yellow pepper, deseeded
    and cut into strips
2–3 shallots, cut into quarters
1 tbsp light olive oil
25 g pitted black or green olives
A handful of rocket
Salt and freshly ground black
    pepper, to taste

FOR THE PIZZA BASE

125 g chickpea (gram) flour
2 tsp olive oil
½ tsp baking powder
¼ tsp salt
300 ml water

FOR THE PESTO SAUCE

A large bunch of basil, chopped
½ avocado, peeled and pitted
25 g pine nuts
Juice of ½ lemon
1 garlic clove, finely chopped
1–2 tbsp nutritional yeast
    (optional)
Salt and freshly ground black
    pepper, to taste

Preheat the oven to 200°C/fan 180°C/gas mark 6.

Arrange the courgettes, pepper and shallots in a baking tray. Drizzle with olive oil and season with salt and freshly ground black pepper; toss until they are coated with oil. Roast in the oven for 20 minutes until slightly charred at the edges.

Make the pizza base while the vegetables are roasting: place the chickpea flour, olive oil, baking powder and salt in a bowl. Gradually whisk in the water until you have a smooth, thick batter. Pour the mixture into a 23-cm non-stick round pizza tin. Bake for 13–15 minutes until the pizza base has set.

Meanwhile, make the pesto by placing all the ingredients in the bowl of a high-speed blender or food processor. Blitz until you have a smooth sauce.

When the pizza base is cooked, spread the pesto over the surface, arrange the roasted vegetables on top and scatter with olives. Serve immediately, garnished with the rocket.

NUTRITION per serving | **556** cals | **22** g protein | **30** g fat (**4** g saturates) | **43** g carbs (**8** g total sugars) | **13** g fibre

Edamame and chickpea falafels

············

These protein-packed falafels are easy to make and perfect for weekend lunches and picnics. They are made with three protein sources – chickpeas, edamame beans and tahini – so are a brilliant way of getting all your amino acids, along with lots of fibre, iron, vitamin E and magnesium. The addition of the edamame beans makes the falafels deliciously moist, so, unlike most bought varieties, they will not turn crumbly when you bite into them.

PART 2 • RECIPES

SERVES 4
MAKES 12 FALAFELS

125 g edamame beans (defrosted, if frozen)
400 g can chickpeas, drained and rinsed
½ medium onion, roughly chopped
60 g tahini
2-cm piece fresh root ginger, peeled and grated
2 garlic cloves, crushed
A handful of fresh coriander, chopped
1 tsp each: ground cumin and ground coriander
½ tsp sweet paprika or a pinch of chilli flakes (depending on taste!)
1 tbsp chickpea (gram) or plain flour
Juice of ½ lemon
½–1 tsp salt
2 tbsp olive oil

TO SERVE

4 wholemeal pittas and ½ quantity Beetroot and Horseradish Hummus (p. 188)
Leafy salad and lemon wedges

Place all the falafel ingredients except the oil in the bowl of a food processor and process until a rough paste forms. It should still have a chunky texture (you don't want to make hummus!). Form the mixture into balls about the size of a walnut. You should be able to make 12.

Heat the oil in a non-stick pan and add the falafels (you may need to do this in two batches). After browning on one side, about 2 minutes, flip them over gently and brown on the other side. Remove with a slotted spoon.

Serve with warmed wholemeal pittas, Beetroot and Horseradish Hummus, a leafy salad and lemon wedges.

NUTRITION per serving (3 falafels)	294 cals | 13 g protein | 19 g fat (3 g saturates) | 15 g carbs (2 g total sugars) | 7 g fibre
	3 falafels, 1 pitta, 1 tbsp Beetroot and Horseradish Hummus and a leafy salad:
	496 cals | 20 g protein | 22 g fat (3 g saturates) | 49 g carbs (4 g total sugars) | 13 g fibre

Tofu satay skewers

·············

Tofu is a brilliant food for vegan athletes as it is rich in protein and calcium, containing high amounts of all nine essential amino acids. Here, I have combined it with a tasty Asian-inspired satay sauce and colourful vegetables. The peanut butter in the sauce adds extra protein, along with fibre and zinc, which is important for healthy immunity. Peppers are packed with vitamin C and other phytonutrients that promote recovery and reduce inflammation. You can substitute whole mushrooms, cherry tomatoes or aubergine slices if you prefer.

SERVES 4
MAKES 8 SKEWERS

320 g marinated tofu pieces*
1 red and 1 green pepper, deseeded and cut into 2-cm squares
8 shallots, halved
2 courgettes, cut into 2-cm slices
Olive or rapeseed oil for brushing

FOR THE SATAY SAUCE

80 g smooth peanut butter
1 tbsp tamari (Japanese soy sauce) or soya sauce
Juice of ½ lime
1 tbsp maple syrup
150 ml canned coconut milk
4 tbsp water
1 garlic clove, crushed
A pinch of dried chilli flakes

TO SERVE

200 g basmati rice and a leafy green salad

Soak 8 wooden skewers in a bowl of warm water for a few minutes (this helps to prevent them burning).

Meanwhile, preheat a grill or barbecue to medium.

Prepare the satay sauce by adding all the ingredients to the bowl of a blender and process until smooth. Add a splash of water if you prefer a thinner sauce. Transfer to a saucepan and warm over a gentle heat. Keep warm while you assemble the tofu skewers.

Thread the tofu cubes and vegetables alternately onto the skewers. Brush with a little oil and cook under the grill or over the barbecue for 5–10 minutes, turning regularly to prevent the kebabs from burning. Serve with the warm satay sauce, cooked rice and salad.

*If using plain tofu, mix together 1 tablespoon tamari (Japanese soy sauce) or soy sauce, 2 tablespoons water and 1 crushed garlic clove in a bowl. Toss the tofu cubes in the mixture and set aside for at least 1 hour to marinate, turning occasionally.

NUTRITION per serving	431 cals	22 g protein	31 g fat (10 g saturates)	13 g carbs (11 g total sugars)	7 g fibre
	Including 50 g (dry weight) rice:				
	611 cals	26 g protein	31 g fat (10 g saturates)	53 g carbs (11 g total sugars)	7 g fibre

Lentil and mushroom no-meatballs in tomato sauce

·············

Crisp on the outside and soft in the middle, these tasty no-meatballs are a healthy substitute for the original version. They are made with lentils and walnuts, so are high in protein, fibre, iron and zinc. You can swap the lentils for canned black beans if you wish. I have added walnuts in this recipe as they are rich in omega-3 fats and supply extra protein, but you can easily swap for Brazils or pecans. Leftover balls can be wrapped in foil and kept in the fridge for up to three days or in the freezer for up to a month.

SERVES 4, MAKES 20 BALLS

1 tbsp ground flaxseed mixed
    with 3 tbsp cold water
2 tbsp light olive or rapeseed oil
1 small onion, finely chopped
2 garlic cloves, chopped
150 g button mushrooms, roughly
    chopped
½ red pepper, deseeded and
    roughly chopped
1 carrot, roughly chopped
1 tsp Italian seasoning (or dried
    oregano)
A handful of fresh coriander or flat-
    leaf parsley, roughly chopped
½ tsp dried chilli flakes, optional
1 tbsp tomato purée
400 g can green or brown lentils,
    drained and rinsed
50 g rolled oats
50 g chopped walnuts
1 tbsp nutritional yeast (optional)
Salt and freshly ground black
    pepper, to taste

FOR THE TOMATO SAUCE

1 tbsp olive oil
1 small onion, finely chopped
2 garlic cloves
2 x 400 g cans chopped tomatoes
1 tbsp tomato purée
½ tsp balsamic vinegar
1 tsp dried oregano

Preheat the oven to 200°C/fan 180°C/gas mark 6 and line a baking tray with baking paper.

Heat 1 tablespoon of the oil in a non-stick frying pan over a low heat. Add the onion and fry for 2–3 minutes, then add the garlic and mushrooms; continue cooking for 5–6 minutes.

Tip the onion and mushroom mixture into the bowl of a food processor. Add the remaining meatball ingredients and pulse a few times until the mixture just comes together when pressed but is still a bit chunky. Alternatively, place in a large mixing bowl and mash together with a potato masher until well combined. Season with salt and freshly ground black pepper.

Make 20 small balls of this mixture by taking tablespoonfuls to roll with clean, moist hands. Arrange the balls on the lined baking tray, brush with the remaining oil and bake in the oven for about 20 minutes – you want them a little crisp on the outside and still soft in the middle.

While the meatballs are cooking, make the tomato sauce. Heat the olive oil in a non-stick pan over a low heat, add the onion and cook for about 5 minutes until softened. Add the garlic and cook for another minute, then add the canned tomatoes, tomato purée, balsamic and oregano. Season with salt and pepper and simmer for about 10–15 minutes until the sauce has thickened.

Add the meatballs to the sauce and serve with pasta and freshly torn basil on top.

TO SERVE

300 g spaghetti or any other variety
    of pasta (cooked according to
    packet instructions)
A handful of fresh basil leaves

NUTRITION per serving	Including 75 g (dry weight) pasta: **648** cals | **23** g protein | **21** g fat (**3** g saturates) | **84** g carbs (**15** g total sugars) | **14** g fibre

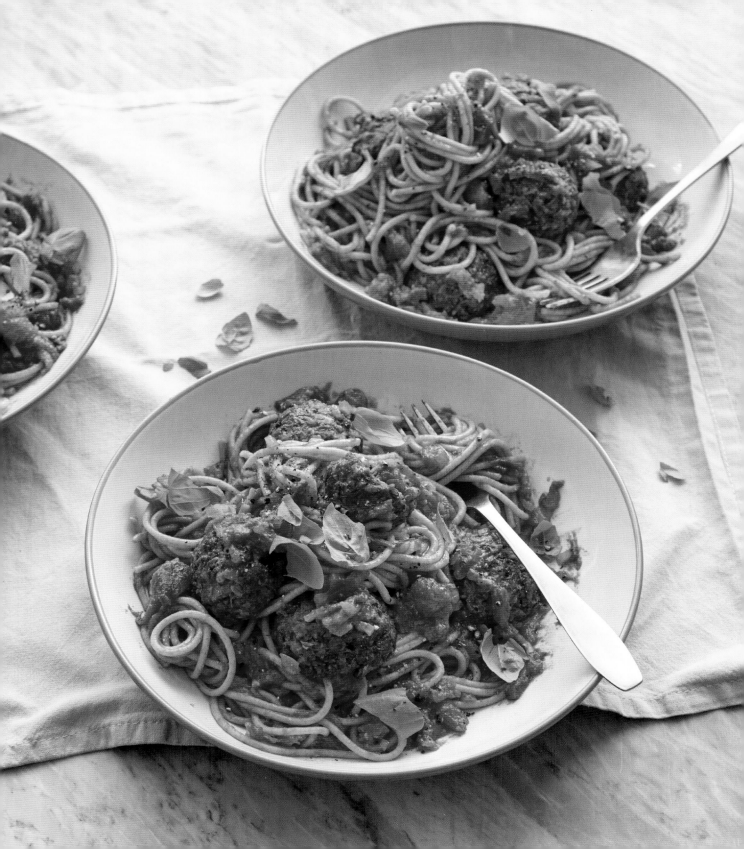

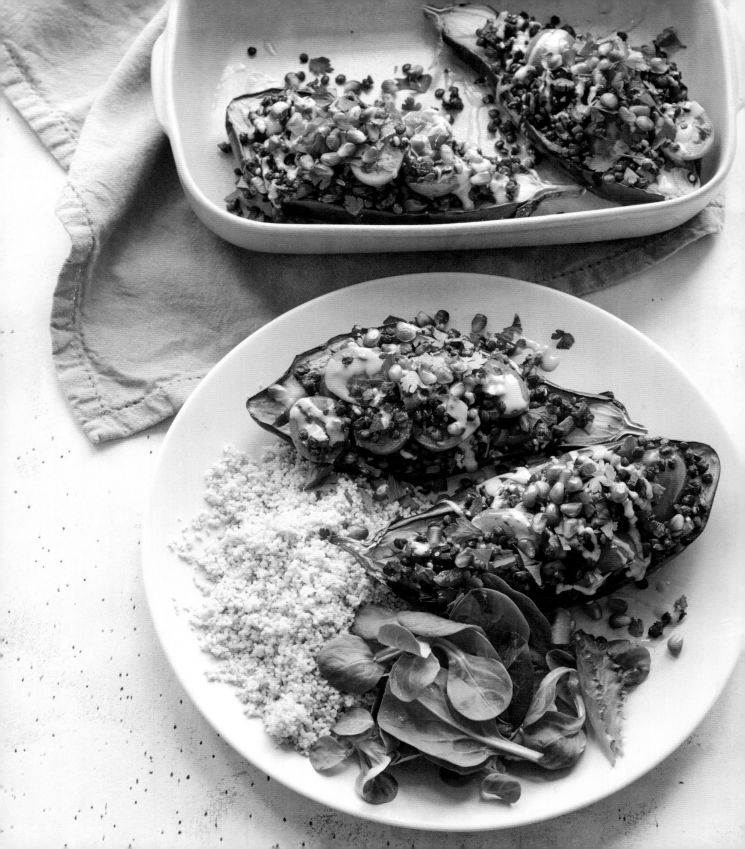

Moroccan lentil-stuffed aubergines with tahini

. . . .

In this healthy, flavour-packed dish, aubergines take centre stage. They are roasted and stuffed with Moroccan-spiced lentils, which is an excellent source of protein, fibre, carbohydrate, iron and zinc. Aubergines are rich in antioxidant phytochemicals, specifically nasunin, which gives the skin its purple hue and protects cells from damage by free radicals during exercise. They are topped with creamy tahini, which provides additional protein plus calcium and healthy fat.

SERVES 2

2 small aubergines
2 tbsp olive oil, plus extra for brushing
1 small onion, finely chopped
1 small red pepper, deseeded and finely chopped
1–2 garlic cloves, crushed
1 tsp ras el hanout
Juice of ½ lemon
250 g pouch-cooked Puy lentils (or 400 g can green or brown lentils)
100 g baby plum tomatoes, halved
Salt and freshly ground black pepper, to taste

TO SERVE

2 tbsp tahini
25 g pomegranate seeds
A small handful of fresh chopped parsley
200 g wholegrain couscous (cooked according to packet instructions) and a leafy salad

Preheat the oven to 200°C/fan 180°C/gas mark 6. Meanwhile, brush a baking tray with a little olive oil.

Slice the aubergines in half lengthways and leave the stem intact. Using a sharp knife, score the flesh side 1 cm deep in a criss-cross diagonal pattern. Transfer to the baking tray, cut side up. Drizzle over 1 tablespoon of the oil and roast in the oven for 25 minutes until the flesh is soft.

Meanwhile, heat the remaining 1 tablespoon of the oil in a non-stick frying pan and fry the onion for 5 minutes until translucent. Add the red pepper, garlic, ras el hanout, lemon juice, salt and freshly ground black pepper; continue cooking for another minute. Stir in the lentils and tomatoes and cook for a further 5 minutes.

Once the aubergines are cooked, remove from the oven (leave the oven on) and allow to cool for a few minutes before scooping out some of the flesh into a bowl (leave enough aubergine flesh so the shell is sturdy enough to hold the lentils). Chop the flesh and add to the lentil mixture. Spoon the mixture into the aubergine halves. Cover loosely in foil and return to the oven for 5 minutes to heat through.

To serve, drizzle over the tahini and scatter over the pomegranate seeds and parsley. Serve with cooked wholegrain couscous and a leafy salad.

NUTRITION per serving	469 cals | 20 g protein | 23 g fat (4 g saturates) | 36 g carbs (12 g total sugars) | 18 g fibre
	Including 50 g (dry weight) wholegrain couscous: 626 cals | 26 g protein | 25 g fat (4 g saturates) | 65 g carbs (14 g total sugars) | 22 g fibre

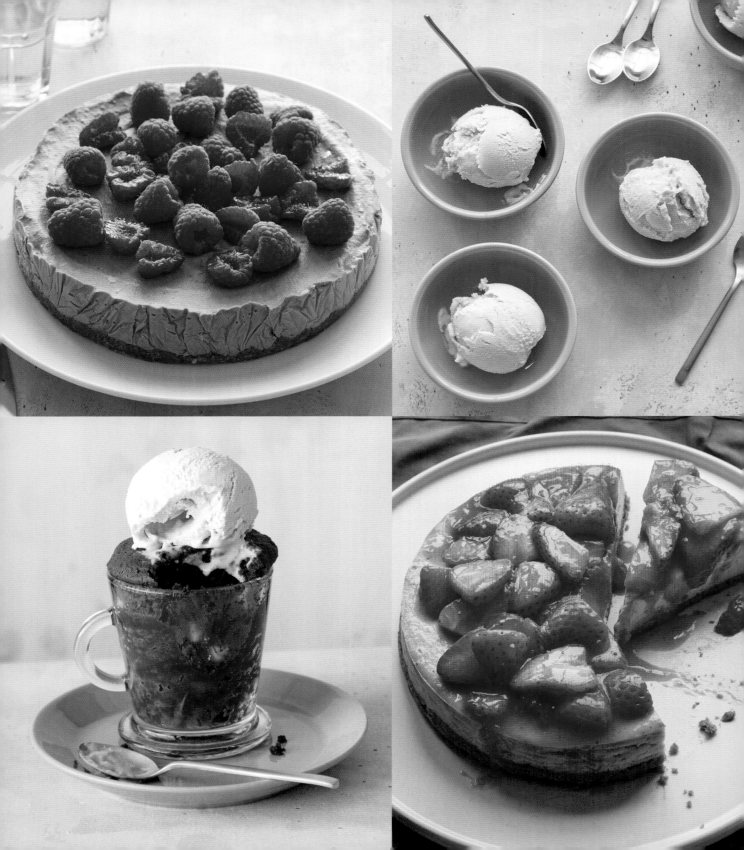

13

Desserts

Clockwise from top left: Raspberry semi-freddo tart;
Vanilla coconut ice cream; Baked lemon cheesecake
with strawberry sauce; Protein chocolate mug cake.

Baked lemon cheesecake with strawberry sauce

· · · · · · · · · · · · ·

This gorgeous New York-style cheesecake is rich in protein and calcium. Made from tofu and cashew nuts in place of soft cheese, it has a rich, creamy texture akin to the traditional dairy version. The key is to soak the cashews beforehand so they blend easily to a smooth paste. The cornflour and tofu both act as an egg replacement, helping the cheesecake 'set' when baked in the oven. The sweet strawberry topping balances the lemony cheesecake perfectly but you can substitute other berries, such as blueberries, blackberries or raspberries if you prefer.

SERVES 8

150 g cashews, soaked overnight
   (or in boiling water for 1 hour)
300 g silken tofu (*see* p. 61)
25 g cornflour
Zest of 1 lemon and juice of
   3 lemons
100 ml agave or maple syrup

FOR THE BASE

100 g wholemeal digestives (or
   your favourite vegan biscuits)
40 g dairy-free spread, melted

FOR THE
STRAWBERRY SAUCE

1½ tsp cornflour
1½ tbsp water
250 g strawberries (fresh or
   frozen), hulled and thickly
   sliced
1–2 tbsp sugar
2 tsp lemon juice

Preheat the oven to 160°C/fan 140°C/gas mark 3. Meanwhile, line the base and sides of a 18-cm springform cake tin with baking paper.

For the base, blitz the biscuits in a food processor until you have fine crumbs, then add the dairy-free spread and pulse until combined. Press the mixture into the bottom of the prepared tin.

For the cheesecake filling, place all the ingredients in a food processor and process until smooth. You may need to scrape down the sides of the bowl a few times. Pour the filling over the biscuit base, smooth the surface with a knife and bake for 40–45 minutes until just set with a slight wobble (it should be creamy on top with just a slight golden hint round the edges). Turn off the oven, prop open the door so that it is slightly ajar and leave the cheesecake to cool inside (this prevents it cracking).

Once cool, remove the cheesecake from the oven. Allow to cool completely before removing from the tin and keep in the fridge for at least two hours before serving.

To make the strawberry sauce, dissolve the cornflour in 1½ tablespoons water. Place the cornflour mixture, strawberries, sugar and lemon juice in a small pan over a low heat. Bring to the boil and simmer for 5 minutes or until the sauce has thickened, stirring continually. Transfer to a bowl and leave to cool. When you are ready to serve, pour the sauce over the cheesecake.

NUTRITION per serving	**291** cals	**8** g protein	**16** g fat (**4** g saturates)	**29** g carbs (**17** g total sugars)	**3** g fibre

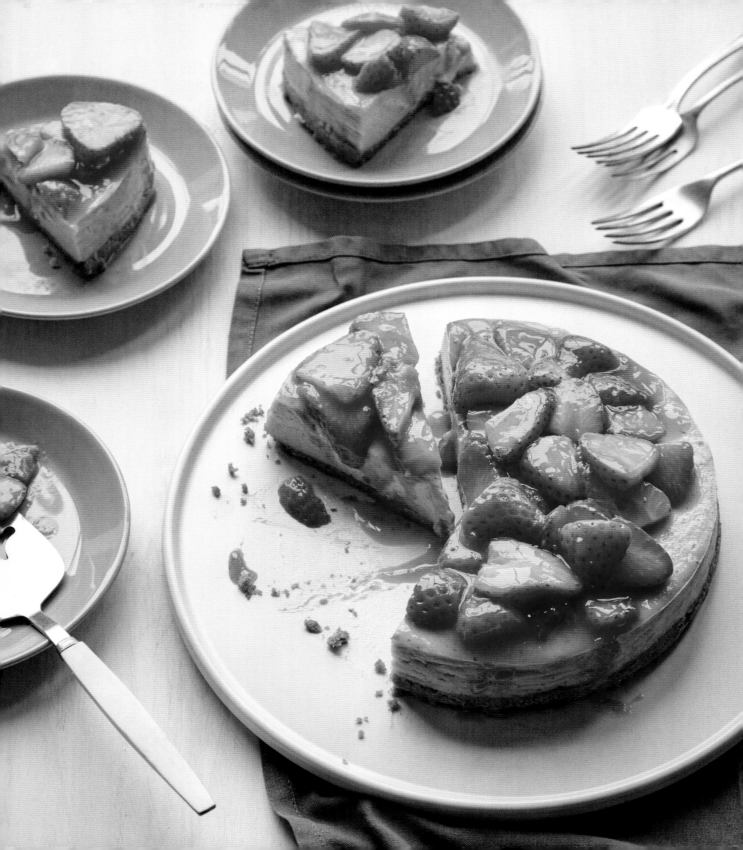

Plum, pear and walnut crumble

....

Plums are loaded with anthocyanins, the pigments that are responsible for the glorious deep purple colour. They have powerful anti-inflammatory and antioxidant properties, which benefit muscle recovery and adaptation following exercise. Adding walnuts to the crumble topping not only gives this crumble a bit of crunch but also increases the content of omega-3 fats, fibre and protein. When plums are not in season, substitute frozen blackberries or blueberries.

SERVES 4

4 ripe purple plums, pitted and quartered
2 Conference pears, peeled, cored and diced (or any other variety)
1 tsp ground cinnamon
Juice of ½ lemon
25 g brown sugar
2 tbsp water

FOR THE CRUMBLE

50 g plain flour
40 g brown sugar
75 g jumbo oats
50 g dairy-free spread
50 g walnuts, roughly chopped

TO SERVE

Soya or coconut yogurt alternative

Preheat the oven to 190°C/fan 170°C/gas mark 5.

To make the fruit filling, place the plums, pears, cinnamon, lemon juice and sugar in a large saucepan with 2 tablespoons water. Bring to the boil, cover and simmer for 10 minutes until the fruit has just softened. Transfer to a 2-litre ovenproof dish.

To prepare the crumble, place the flour, brown sugar and oats in a mixing bowl. Add the dairy-free spread and rub into the mixture until it resembles breadcrumbs. Alternatively, mix together in a food mixer. Stir in the chopped walnuts.

Scatter the crumble topping over the fruit and bake for 15–20 minutes until golden and bubbling around the edges. Serve with soya or coconut yogurt alternative.

NUTRITION per serving | **395** cals | **6** g protein | **17** g fat (**3** g saturates) | **51** g carbs (**28** g total sugars) | **6** g fibre

Strawberry frozen yogurt

. . . .

This highly nutritious dessert made with frozen fruit provides your entire daily requirement for vitamin C. This vitamin helps to protect cells from oxidative damage caused by free radicals during intense exercise as well as to make collagen, the main protein in tendons, bones, ligaments and cartilage. Feel free to swap the strawberries for other frozen fruits, such as peaches, raspberries, pineapple or mangos.

SERVES 4

600 g frozen strawberries
3 tbsp agave nectar or icing sugar
125 g plain Greek-style soya
   yogurt alternative (or coconut
   yogurt alternative)
1 tbsp lemon juice

Place the frozen strawberries, agave nectar (or icing sugar), yogurt alternative and lemon juice in the bowl of a food processor. Process until creamy, about five minutes.

Serve the frozen yogurt immediately or transfer to an airtight container and store it in the freezer for up to 1 month.

NUTRITION per serving | **112** cals | **3** g protein | **2** g fat (**<1** g saturates) | **18** g carbs (**18** g total sugars) | **6** g fibre

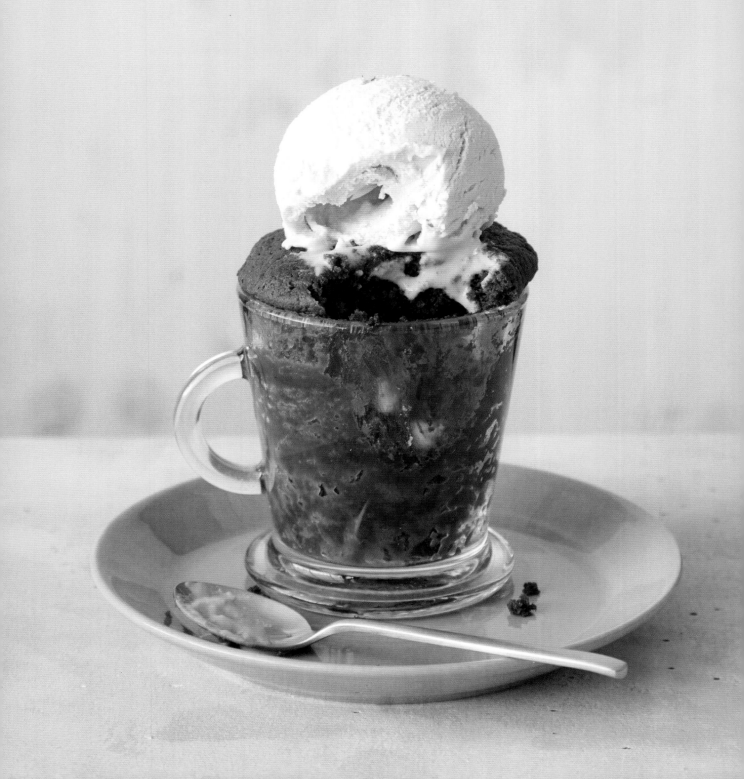

Protein chocolate mug cake

. . . .

A mug cake is literally a single serving cake, made in a mug and cooked in the microwave. It takes literally minutes to make, so is perfect when you want an impromptu dessert or snack. Made with vegan protein powder, one serving gives you 24 g protein, the ideal amount for muscle recovery. However, you can omit the protein powder if you don't have any – it will still taste delicious! It also contains almond butter and ground almonds, which give the cake a super-fudgy and brownie-like texture, plus healthy fats and vitamin E. Feel free to substitute chopped walnuts or pecans for the chocolate chips.

SERVES 1

30 g plain flour
½ tsp baking powder
1 tbsp cacao or cocoa powder
1 tbsp chocolate vegan protein
   powder
1 tbsp brown sugar or maple
   syrup
Pinch of salt
1 tbsp almond butter or light
   olive or rapeseed oil
5 tbsp almond milk alternative
½ tsp vanilla extract
1 tbsp ground almonds
1 tbsp dark chocolate chips or
   cacao nibs

TO SERVE

Vegan vanilla ice cream or
coconut yogurt alternative

Mix together the flour, baking powder, cacao or cocoa powder, protein powder, sugar or maple syrup and salt in a microwave-safe mug. This cake will rise by about one third in the microwave so make sure the mug is high enough.

Add the nut butter or oil, almond milk alternative, vanilla extract, ground almonds and chocolate chips; whisk with a fork until you have a smooth batter. Microwave on full power (800W) for 1 minute 30 seconds. All microwaves vary, so you may need a little less or more cooking time, depending on your microwave model. Start with a shorter time, then check and cook the cake a little longer in 15-second intervals until the surface is not sticky anymore and just firm to the touch. Leave to cool for a few minutes, then serve with vegan vanilla ice cream or coconut yogurt alternative.

NUTRITION per serving* | **483** cals | **24** g protein | **19** g fat (**4** g saturates) | **50** g carbs (**22** g total sugars) | **8** g fibre

*without ice cream or yogurt

Raspberry semi-freddo tart

....

A semi-freddo is a mousse-like dessert that is served half-frozen. The traditional recipe with whipped cream and egg yolks is high in saturated fat but my version made with cashews and coconut yogurt alternative (I used Koko) served on a crunchy biscuit base is gloriously light, tangy, fruity and delicious. It is low in saturated fat, high in protein, vitamin C and healthy fats. If you don't have fresh raspberries, then frozen fruit works equally well. The key is to serve it when it is in a semi-frozen state.

SERVES 8

250 g cashews, soaked in water overnight (or in boiling water for 1 hour)
2 tbsp lemon juice
250 g coconut yogurt alternative
150 g fresh raspberries
100 g icing sugar

FOR THE BASE

100 g wholemeal digestive biscuits (or your favourite vegan biscuit)
40 g almonds
40 g dairy-free spread, melted

FOR THE TOPPING (OPTIONAL)

100 g fresh raspberries

Line a 20-cm springform cake tin with cling film.

To make the base, blitz the biscuits and almonds in a food processor, then add the melted dairy-free spread and pulse until combined. Press the mixture into the base of the cake tin. Pop in the freezer while you make the filling.

Rinse and drain the cashews and add to the food processor, along with the lemon juice; process for 2–3 minutes until smooth (depending on the power of your processor). You may need to stop and scrape down the sides with a spatula a couple of times. Then add the coconut yogurt alternative, raspberries and icing sugar. Blitz until smooth, then pour on top of the base of the cheesecake. Smooth with a knife. Place back in the freezer and leave to freeze for a few hours or overnight.

Remove from the freezer about 3 hours before serving and place in the fridge. When ready to serve, remove the cheesecake from the tin and place on a plate. Top with fresh raspberries, if liked. Keep any leftovers in the freezer for up to three months.

NUTRITION per serving | **383** cals | **9** g protein | **25** g fat (**6** g saturates) | **30** g carbs (**18** g total sugars) | **3** g fibre

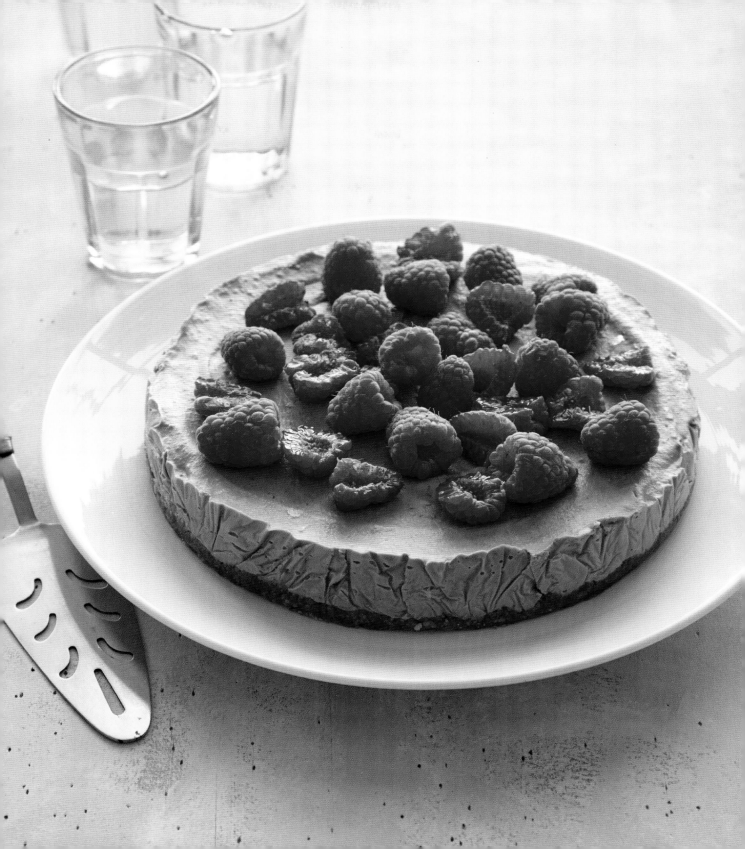

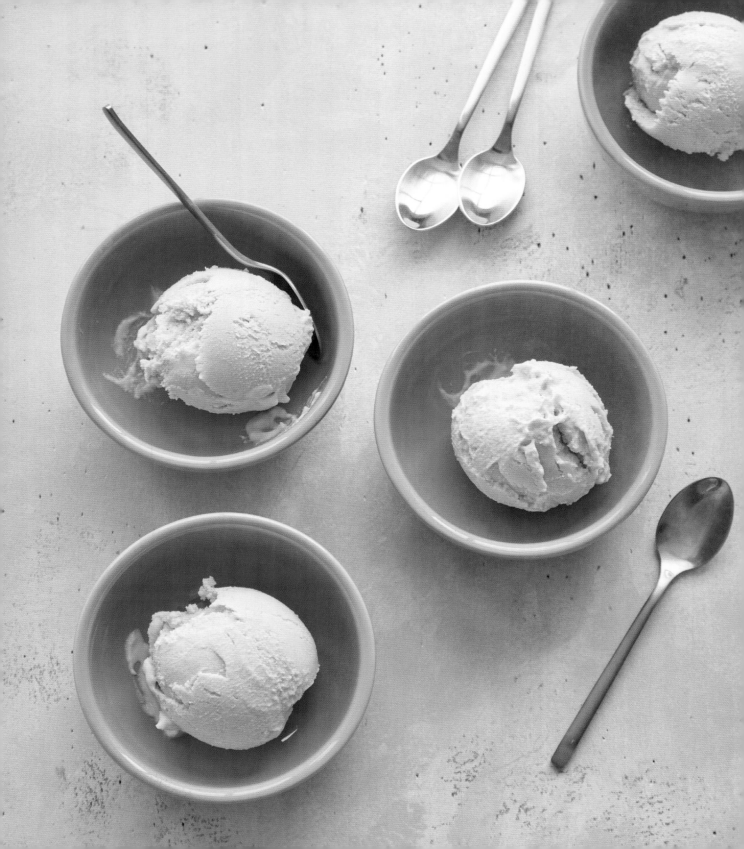

Vanilla coconut ice cream

. . . .

This gorgeous vegan ice cream made with cashews and coconut cream is packed with nutrients and has all the richness, flavour and creaminess of the dairy version. It provides protein, fibre, iron, thiamin, magnesium and zinc. I use this recipe as a base to make lots of other flavours: for raspberry ice cream, add 150 g raspberries to the blender; for chocolate ice cream, add one tablespoon of cacao or cocoa powder. You won't need an ice cream machine for this recipe, although it will be slightly creamier if you do use one.

SERVES 8

150 g cashews, soaked in water
   overnight (or in boiling water
   for 1 hour), drained and rinsed
300 ml coconut cream
2 tsp vanilla paste (or vanilla
   extract)
2 tbsp agave or maple syrup,
   or icing sugar

Place the cashews, coconut cream, vanilla paste and agave or maple syrup or icing sugar in the bowl of a high-power blender and blitz until completely smooth – about 3 minutes.

Transfer to a freezer-safe container, place in the freezer and just before it is frozen, bring it out and mix it again with a fork. This will help prevent ice crystals forming and produce a smooth texture. Return to the freezer and freeze overnight or until firm.

Take out of the freezer for 20 minutes before serving.

Alternatively, if you have an ice cream machine, pour the mixture into the bowl and churn according to the manufacturer's instructions.

NUTRITION per serving | **208** cals | **4** g protein | **17** g fat (**9** g saturates) | **9** g carbs (**6** g total sugars) | **1** g fibre

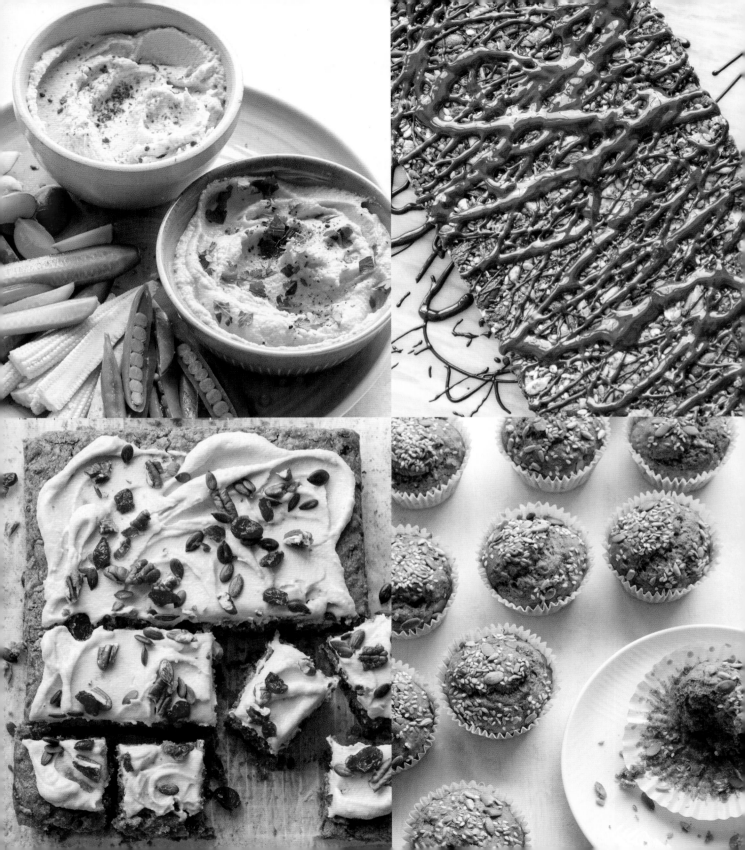

CHAPTER

14

Snacks

Clockwise from top left: Hummus – three ways;
Super-seedy bars; Seeded banana muffins;
Carrot cake traybake with cashew frosting.

Almond and chocolate chip energy bites

· · · · · · · · · · · · ·

These tasty energy bites require no baking and are a brilliant snack for long endurance workouts. Made with oats, dried fruit and nuts, they provide a perfect combination of carbohydrate, protein and healthy fat to sustain your energy levels. I recommend wrapping them individually in cling film or foil, which you can then pop in your pocket, running belt, or kit bag. For a change, you can swap the almonds for desiccated coconut or any other nuts you fancy, or swap the almond butter for peanut butter.

MAKES 24

125 g rolled oats
50 g dark chocolate chips
50 g flaked or chopped almonds
50 g raisins
25 g runny honey
125 g almond butter
1 tsp vanilla extract

In a mixing bowl, combine the oats, chocolate chips, almonds and raisins.

Add the remaining ingredients and mix until the mixture begins to clump together and forms a sticky ball. You can do this by hand or using a food mixer.

Turn the mixture out and press or roll between two sheets of cling film to 1 cm thickness. Transfer to the fridge for 30 minutes or so until firm. Peel off the cling film and cut into 24 small squares. Alternatively, roll into bitesize balls. Store in an airtight container in the fridge for up to five days.

NUTRITION per bite | **88** cals | **3** g protein | **5** g fat (**1** g saturates) | **7** g carbs (**4** g total sugars) | **1** g fibre

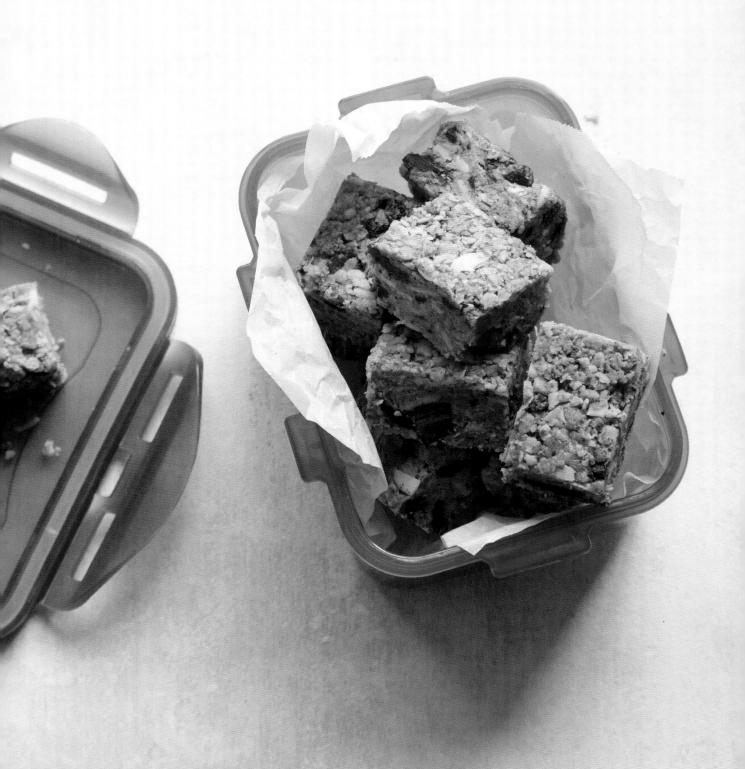

Almond butter cookies

....

These scrumptious cookies are packed with almonds, making them ideal post-exercise snacks. Almonds are nutritional powerhouses, providing plenty of protein, fibre, monounsaturated fats, calcium, iron, zinc, magnesium, B vitamins and vitamin E, a powerful antioxidant that helps protect cells from damage during intense exercise.

MAKES 20

175 g almond butter
75 g dairy-free spread
75 g sugar
25 g golden or agave syrup
75 g ground almonds
125 g self-raising flour
½ tsp vanilla extract
20 whole almonds

Preheat the oven to 190°C/fan 170°C/gas mark 5 and line 2 baking trays with baking paper.

Place all of the ingredients apart from the whole almonds in a large bowl and mix together until you have a smooth dough. Alternatively, use a food mixer.

Roll heaped teaspoons of the mixture into balls about 2-cm diameter. Place on the baking trays about 3 cm apart, press an almond into the top of each ball and flatten lightly with your palm. Bake for 10–12 minutes until light golden. Cool for a few minutes before transferring to a wire rack. They will keep in an airtight tin for up to a week.

NUTRITION per cookie | **148** cals | **4** g protein | **10** g fat (**1** g saturates) | **10** g carbs (**5** g total sugars) | **2** g fibre

Apricot oat bars

. . . .

Tangy apricot compote sandwiched between two layers of glorious oaty flapjack,
these bars make a healthy alternative to shop-bought snack bars. They provide plenty of fibre
and beta-carotene, a powerful antioxidant which promotes recovery after exercise. Substitute
250 g dried apricots and 6 tablespoons water if you don't have fresh apricots.

MAKES 12

6 fresh apricots
2 tbsp water
125 g light brown sugar
200 g dairy-free spread
100 g golden syrup
300 g rolled oats
50 g plain flour
100 g flaked almonds

Preheat the oven to 180°C/fan 160°C/gas mark 4. Meanwhile,
line a 20 cm square tin with baking paper.

To make the filling, place the apricots, water and 25 g of the sugar in
a pan. Heat gently, stirring occasionally until you have a thick purée,
about 10 minutes. Put aside to cool and then mash roughly with
a fork (a few lumps are OK). Leave to cool.

Melt the dairy-free spread with the remaining 100 g sugar and golden
syrup in a pan over a low heat. Stir in the oats, flour and almonds, and
mix well. Press about half of the mixture firmly into the prepared tin.
Spread the filling evenly over the top, then sprinkle the remaining
mixture evenly over the top and press down gently with the back
of a spoon.

Bake for 25–30 minutes until lightly golden. Leave to cool in the
tin before cutting into 12 bars. They will keep in an airtight tin for
up to three days.

NUTRITION per bar | **327** cals | **6** g protein | **16** g fat (**3** g saturates) | **38** g carbs (**18** g total sugars) | **3** g fibre

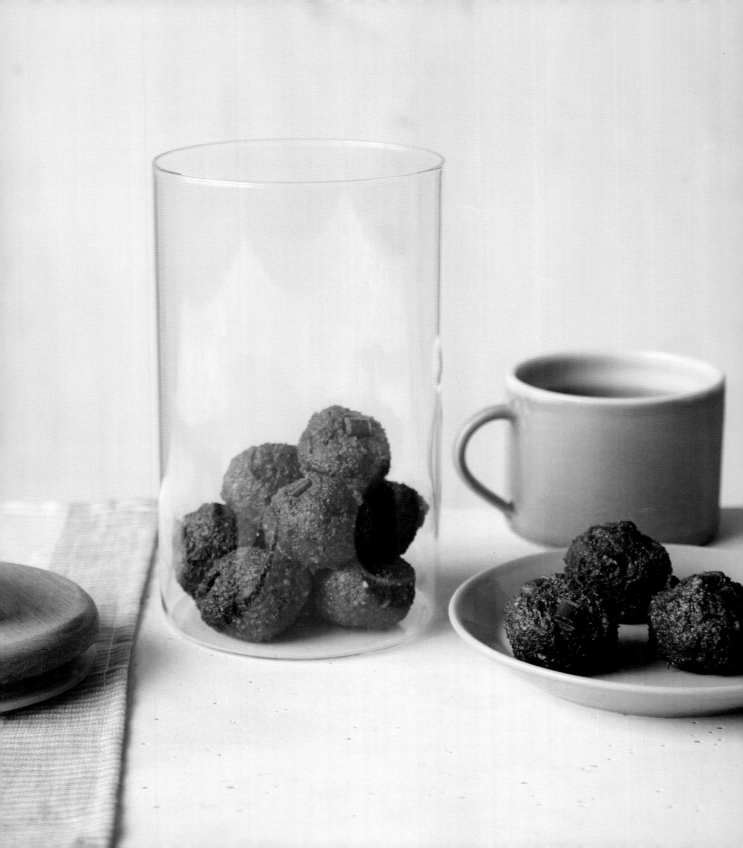

Brownie energy balls

·············

These no-bake energy balls are the perfect fuelling snack when you are exercising hard for longer than an hour. Each one supplies 8 g carbohydrate, along with iron, B vitamins, omega-3s and magnesium. Wrap in cling film or foil, pop in your pocket or belt and aim to consume four per hour (or two every 30 minutes). This will give you 32 g carbohydrate, the amount deemed optimal for maintaining blood glucose levels during exercise (pp. 42–43). You can substitute almonds or hazelnuts for any of the nuts, or dried cherries or cranberries for the chocolate chips.

MAKES 16 BALLS

75 g walnuts
50 g cashews
150 g ready-to-eat soft or
    Medjool dates, pitted*
2 tbsp cacao or cocoa powder
¼ tsp vanilla extract
1 tbsp dark chocolate chips

Place the walnuts, cashews, dates, cacao or cocoa powder and vanilla extract in the bowl of a food processor. Process until the mixture comes together and forms a stiff paste (you may need to scrape down the mixture from the sides of the bowl a few times). Add a little water if the mixture seems too crumbly. Add the chocolate chips and pulse a couple of times.

Form the mixture into 16 balls. Place in a glass storage jar or airtight container and store in the fridge for up to a week, or in the freezer for up to three months.

*Or use standard dried dates: Leave to soak in boiling water for 10–15 minutes, then drain.

NUTRITION per ball | **89** cals | **2** g protein | **5** g fat (**1** g saturates) | **8** g carbs (**6** g total sugars) | **1** g fibre

Carrot cake traybake with cashew frosting

. . . .

Carrot cake has long been a favourite of mine, so I wanted to create a vegan version without eggs and dairy that tasted just as delicious as the traditional cake. Here, I have replaced butter with rapeseed oil, eggs with baking powder and bicarbonate of soda, and used an icing made from cashew nuts. I have also used wholemeal spelt flour (p. 60) instead of white, as it contains almost three times as much fibre and twice as much iron. Ground almonds and grated carrots make the cake extra-moist, while the addition of pumpkin seeds and pecans provides valuable omega-3s. Dried cranberries in place of sultanas deliver an anthocyanin hit, while the cashew icing provides extra protein, fibre and healthy fat.

MAKES 16 SQUARES

Dairy-free spread to grease
250 g wholemeal spelt or
   wheat flour
3 tsp baking powder
1 tsp bicarbonate of soda
2 tsp cinnamon
½ tsp nutmeg
1 tsp ground ginger
125 g sugar
60 g ground almonds
225 ml plant milk alternative
120 ml rapeseed oil
3 carrots, grated
Zest of 1 orange
75 g dried cranberries
75 g pecans, chopped
40 g pumpkin seeds
A few extra cranberries, pecans
   and seeds, to decorate

FOR THE FROSTING

125 g cashews, soaked overnight
   (or in boiling water for 1 hour)
40 g icing sugar or maple syrup
1 tbsp plant milk alternative
1 tsp lemon juice
1 tsp vanilla extract

Preheat the oven to 180°C/fan 160°C/gas mark 4. Meanwhile, grease and line a 25 x 20 cm baking tin with baking paper.

In a large bowl, mix the flour, baking powder, bicarbonate of soda, cinnamon, nutmeg, ginger, sugar and ground almonds. In a separate bowl, whisk together the plant milk alternative and rapeseed oil, then tip them into the large bowl with the dry ingredients. Mix until combined, then fold in the carrots, orange zest, cranberries, pecans and pumpkin seeds. Transfer to the prepared tin, smooth the batter with a spatula and bake for 40 minutes or until a skewer inserted comes out clean and the edges of the cake start to come away from the tin. Cool in the tin on a wire rack.

Meanwhile make the frosting: Blend all the ingredients in a food processor until very smooth. Be patient – this may take a while, depending on your blender. Add an extra splash of milk, if necessary. Chill in the fridge until needed.

Remove the cake from the tin, transfer to a board and spread the icing over the cake. Scatter with extra cranberries, pecans and seeds. The cake will keep for up to two days in an airtight tin, or frozen for up to three months.

NUTRITION per square | **305** cals | **6** g protein | **18** g fat (**2** g saturates) | **27** g carbs (**15** g total sugars) | **3** g fibre

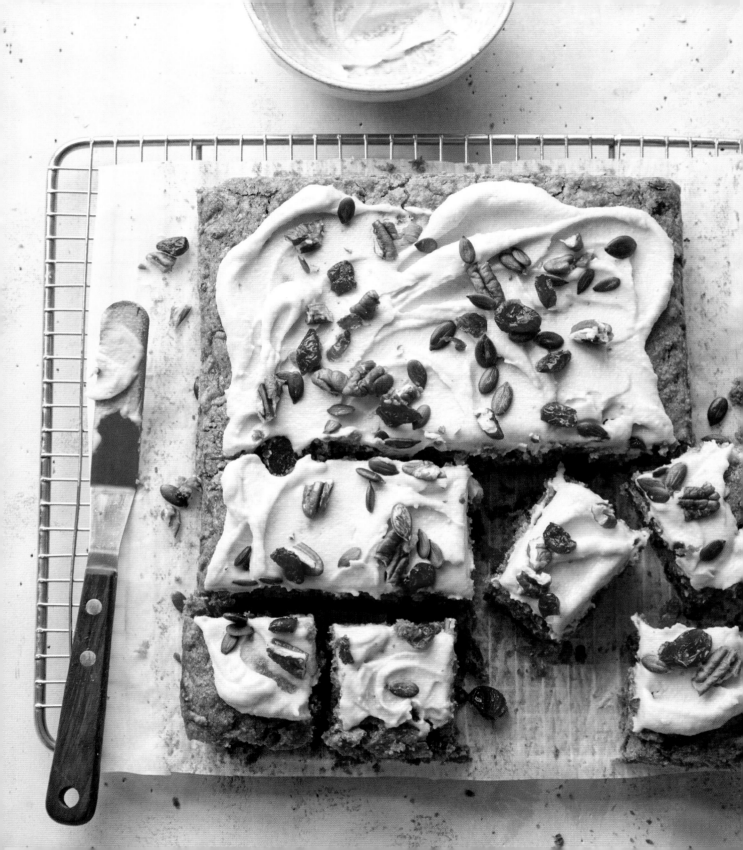

Cashew cream

·············

I admit that I was once dismissive of the merits of cashew cream – it sounded such an unlikely substitute for the real thing. But then I tried making it and suddenly a whole new world of culinary possibilities opened up. It's not only a substitute for dairy cream but it also makes a thick, delicious dip with a creamy consistency similar to mayonnaise, a tasty dressing for roasted vegetables or crunchy salads, or a cooling accompaniment swirled on soup, curry or chilli. Cashews are a great source of heart-healthy unsaturated fats, protein, fibre, B vitamins, vitamin E and magnesium.

MAKES 8 SERVINGS

FOR SAVOURY CASHEW CREAM

150 g unsalted cashews
300 ml, plus 120 ml water
A pinch of salt
1 tbsp nutritional yeast flakes
1 tsp lemon juice
A pinch of cayenne pepper (optional)

FOR SWEET CASHEW CREAM

150 g unsalted cashews
300 ml, plus 120 ml water
1 Medjool date (or 2 tbsp maple syrup)
A few drops of vanilla extract (optional)

To make the savoury cashew cream: place the cashews in a medium bowl and cover with 300 ml water. Set aside uncovered at room temperature for several hours, preferably overnight. They should break apart when pressed between two fingers.

Drain the cashews, then tip them with the nutritional yeast, lemon juice and cayenne pepper (if using), with 120 ml water and salt into a blender. If you want a thinner cream, use a little more water.

Blend on high speed until completely smooth, about 3 minutes, stopping to scrape down the sides of the blender at least once.

To make the sweet cashew cream: place the cashews and date (if using) in a medium bowl and cover with 300 ml water. Set aside uncovered at room temperature for several hours, preferably overnight. They should break apart when pressed between two fingers.

Drain the cashews, then tip them with the date into a blender with 120 ml water. If you want a thinner cream, use a little more water. Add the maple syrup and vanilla, if using.

Blend on high speed until completely smooth, about 3 minutes, stopping to scrape down the sides of the blender at least once.

Use immediately or transfer to an airtight container and refrigerate for up to a week.

NUTRITION per 1 table-spoon (30 g) | **74** cals | **3** g protein | **6** g fat (**1** g saturates) | **2** g carbs (**1** g total sugars) | **1** g fibre

Chickpea and sesame seed crackers

. . . .

These protein-rich crackers are a nutritious alternative to ordinary crackers and make excellent savoury pre- or post-exercise snacks, either on their own or spread with hummus or nut butter. They are made with chickpea (gram) flour, which is essentially ground chickpeas. It is significantly higher in protein and fibre than wheat flour, which makes it a worthwhile addition to your vegan larder. You can swap the sesame seeds for flax or sunflower seeds, za'atar or fresh rosemary, if you prefer.

MAKES APPROXIMATELY 24

150 g chickpea (gram) flour
A pinch of paprika (optional)
1 tsp baking powder
1 tbsp black sesame seeds
½ tsp salt
2 tbsp extra virgin olive or rapeseed oil
3–4 tbsp water

Preheat the oven to 180°C/fan 160°C/gas mark 4.

In a bowl, combine the chickpea (gram) flour, paprika, baking powder, black sesame seeds and salt. Mix in the oil and then slowly add the water until the mixture comes together and a dough ball is formed. If it is dry, add a little more water. Knead until smooth.

Roll out the dough as thinly and evenly as possible between two pieces of baking paper, remove the top paper layer, then slice the dough into small rectangles or triangles. Carefully transfer the baking paper onto a baking tray.

Bake in the oven for 12–15 minutes, or until golden and crispy. The crackers will keep in an airtight container for up to three days.

NUTRITION per cracker | **32** cals | **2** g protein | **2** g fat (<**1** g saturates) | **3** g carbs (<**1** g total sugars) | **1** g fibre

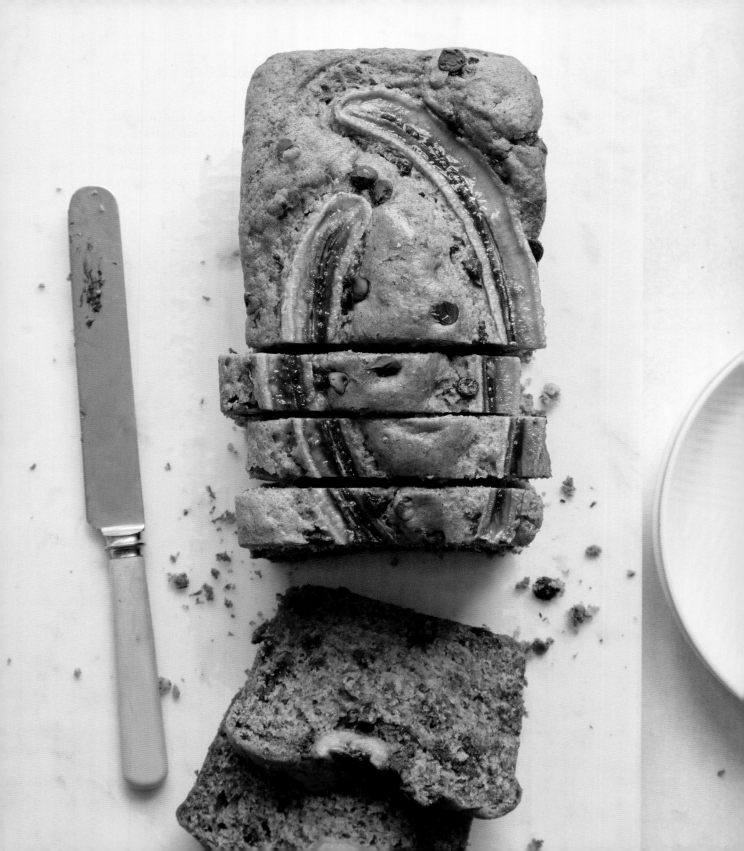

Chocolate chip banana bread

. . . .

Banana bread is such a staple for athletes and one that can be made successfully without eggs. In this recipe I have used ground flaxseed as an egg substitute – its flavour is masked by the bananas. I have also used rapeseed oil, which is low in saturated fat and high in healthy monounsaturated fat. This bread is delicious served warm (you get melted gooey chocolate in each slice) or cold with a generous spoonful of nut butter, especially when the loaf is a few days old. Kept wrapped, it will last for two days at room temperature, or freeze for up to two months.

MAKES 10 SLICES

1 tbsp ground flaxseed
3 tablespoons water
2 ripe bananas, plus 1 banana
    for the top
100 ml light olive or rapeseed oil
3 tbsp plant milk alternative
    (any type)
225 g self-raising flour
2 tsp baking powder
½ tsp salt
1 tsp ground cinnamon
100 g sugar
100 g dark chocolate chips or
    dark chocolate broken into
    pieces

Preheat the oven to 160°C/fan 140°C/gas mark 3. Meanwhile, line a 900 g loaf tin with baking paper.

Mix the ground flaxseed with 3 tablespoons water and leave to stand for 15 minutes.

Peel and mash two of the bananas in a bowl, then stir in the oil and milk alternative. Place the flour, baking powder, salt, cinnamon and sugar in a large mixing bowl or food mixer and mix together. Stir in the mashed banana mixture and flaxseed mixture, then fold in the chocolate chips.

Spoon the mixture into the prepared tin and level the top. Peel and halve the remaining banana lengthways, then place on top of the mixture. Bake for 1 hour until golden on top and springy to the touch in the centre, or until a skewer inserted in the centre comes out clean. Leave in the tin for 15 minutes, then turn out onto a wire rack to cool completely before slicing. It will keep in an airtight tin for up to three days.

VARIATIONS

. . . .

- *Banana muffins:* Divide the mixture between 12 muffin cases and bake at 190°C/fan 170°C/gas mark 5 for 20 minutes.

- *Triple Chocolate:* Add 2 tablespoons cacao or cocoa powder and an extra 2 tablespoons plant milk alternative to the mixture, then stir in 50 g vegan white chocolate pieces and 50 g plain chocolate chips.

- *Banana Walnut:* Replace the chocolate chips with 100 g chopped walnuts.

- *Banana Cranberry:* Replace half the chocolate chips with dried cranberries.

NUTRITION per slice | **273** cals | **3** g protein | **11** g fat (**3** g saturates) | **39** g carbs (**21** g total sugars) | **2** g fibre

Chickpea blondies
with dark chocolate ganache

· · · · · · · · · · · · · ·

Puréed chickpeas make a healthy fibre-rich base for blondies and brownies,
avoiding the requirement for adding fat or oil. Their flavour is masked by the addition
of vanilla and chocolate chips. In this recipe, I have combined them with peanut butter
to achieve that glorious, gooey texture of blondies. However, you can substitute any other
nut butter or tahini, or add chopped pecans instead of the chocolate chips.
Top with a layer of dark chocolate ganache for a decadent treat.

MAKES 16 SQUARES

50 g rolled oats
400 g can chickpeas, drained
    and rinsed
125 g peanut butter (or your
    favourite nut butter)
90 ml agave or maple syrup
3 tbsp plant milk alternative
    (any type)
1–2 tsp vanilla extract
¼ tsp salt
½ tsp baking powder
75 g dark chocolate chips or
    chopped dark chocolate

FOR THE DARK
CHOCOLATE GANACHE
(OPTIONAL)

100 ml canned coconut milk
100 g dark chocolate, coarsely
    chopped

Preheat the oven to 180°C/fan 160°C/gas mark 4. Meanwhile, line a
18 cm square tin with baking paper. Place the oats in the bowl of a food
processor and process for a few seconds until they turn into flour. Then
add all the remaining ingredients except the chocolate chips or chopped
dark chocolate and process until the mixture resembles cookie dough.
You may need to stop and scrape the mixture from the sides of the
food processor with a spatula a couple of times.

Transfer to a bowl, then fold in the chocolate chips, reserving a few for
decoration, then pour into the prepared tin. Smooth the surface with
a knife and sprinkle the reserved chocolate chips on top.

Bake for 20–25 minutes until lightly golden. Leave to cool in the tin
– they will firm up as they cool.

Meanwhile, make the ganache, if liked, by heating the coconut milk in
a small saucepan until almost boiling. Remove from the heat, then add
the chocolate; leave to stand for a few minutes until the chocolate has
melted. Spread over the cooled blondies, then cut into 16 squares.
They will keep in an airtight container for up to three days.

NUTRITION
per blondie | **121** cals | **4** g protein | **6** g fat (**2** g saturates) | **12** g carbs (**7** g total sugars) | **2** g fibre

Including chocolate ganache:
164 cals | **4** g protein | **9** g fat (**4** g saturates) | **16** g carbs (**11** g total sugars) | **2** g fibre

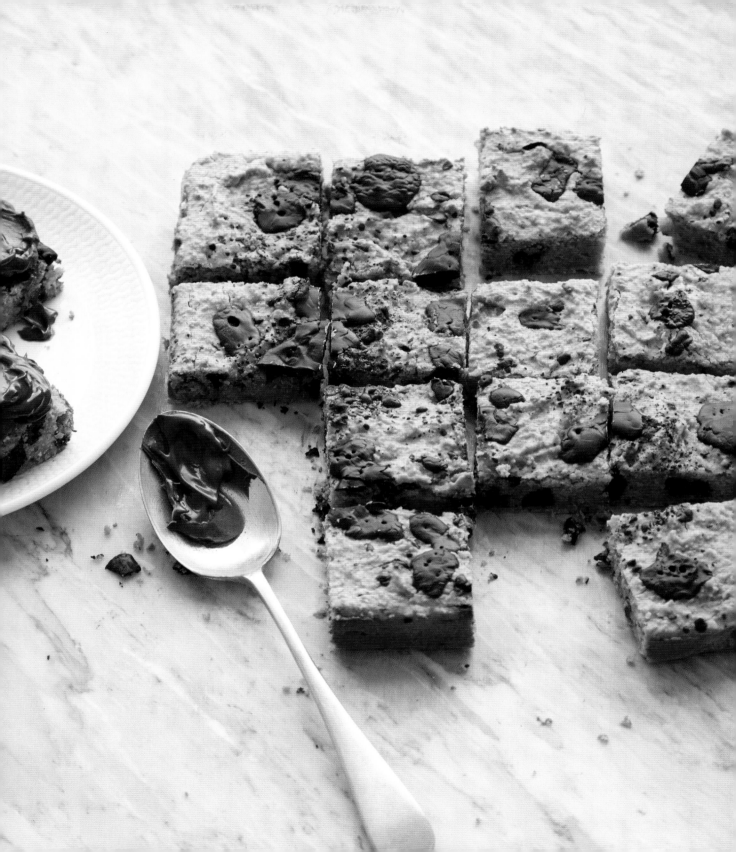

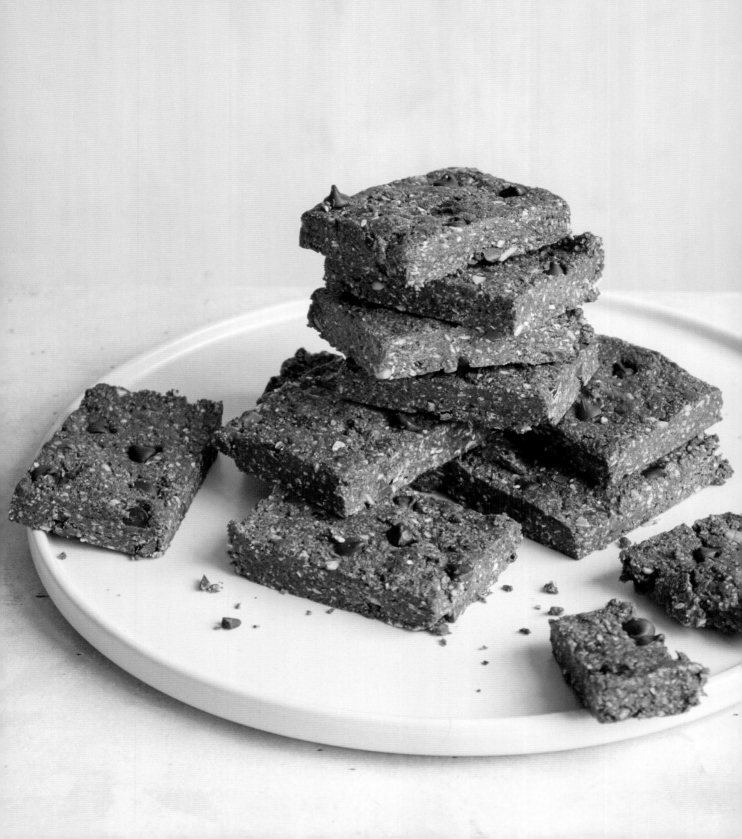

Chocolate protein bars

. . . .

These tasty bars made with vegan protein powder are ideal recovery snacks. Each bar supplies 10 g protein, plus plenty of fibre, B vitamins, vitamin E, calcium and magnesium. Wrap individually in cling film or foil and pop in your kit bag. You can swap the almond butter for your favourite nut butter, or substitute raisins for the chocolate chips if you prefer.

MAKES 12 BARS

125 g rolled oats
125 g almond butter
50 g ground almonds
60 g chocolate vegan protein powder
150 g maple or golden syrup
3 tbsp mixed seeds
½ tsp cinnamon
50 g chocolate chips

Line a 20 cm square tin with baking paper or foil.

Place the oats in the bowl of a food processor and pulse until they are ground into oat flour.

Add the almond butter, ground almonds, protein powder, maple or golden syrup, seeds and cinnamon. Process until the mixture starts to clump together, then add the chocolate chips; pulse just until they are incorporated.

Transfer the mixture to the lined tin, pressing down firmly. Chill in the fridge for at least two hours before slicing into bars. The bars will keep for up to five days in the fridge.

NUTRITION per bar | **229** cals | **9** g protein | **12** g fat (**2** g saturates) | **19** g carbs (**10** g total sugars) | **3** g fibre

Chocummus

....

This delicious, healthy chocolate dip has the luxurious decadence of chocolate spread but with more protein and considerably less sugar and saturated fat. It is perfect on pancakes, toast, porridge or for dipping strawberries, apple slices, banana or salty pretzels.

MAKES 350g

400 g can chickpeas, drained and rinsed
2 tbsp cacao or cocoa powder
2 tbsp tahini or nut butter
2–3 tbsp maple or agave syrup, to taste
½ tsp vanilla extract
A pinch of salt
2 tbsp plant milk alternative (any type)

Place all the ingredients in the bowl of a food processor and pulse until the mixture is smooth and creamy. You may need to stop and scrape the mixture from the sides with a spatula a couple of times. Add a little extra water if you want a thinner consistency. Taste and add extra syrup, if liked. Transfer to bowl or jar and store, covered, in the fridge for up to a week.

NUTRITION per 1 tablespoon (30 g)	**58** cals | **3** g protein
	2 g fat (**<1** g saturates)
	5 g carbs (**2** g total sugars)
	2 g fibre

Kale crisps

....

Making kale crisps is very easy and a healthy alternative to shop-bought snacks. Kale is an extraordinarily rich source of beta-carotene, vitamins C and K, as well as good source of magnesium, potassium and B vitamins. It is worth noting that kale is significantly lower in oxalates than spinach, which means that it does not block the body's uptake of calcium (*see also* pp. 27–28).

SERVES 4

8 large kale leaves
2 tsp olive or rapeseed oil
¼ tsp salt
Seasonings of choice, such as smoked paprika, cumin, chilli powder or nutritional yeast (optional)

Preheat the oven to 150°C/fan 130°C/gas mark 2

Remove the central stem from the kale leaves and tear into large pieces. Place them in a large bowl and rub with the oil so they are well-coated. Sprinkle with salt and, if you like, your favourite seasonings, then arrange on a baking tray in a single layer.

Bake for about 20 minutes or until crispy but still green – watch closely as they can burn easily. Remove from the oven and leave to cool. They will crisp up more as they cool down. Best when fresh, but they can be stored in an airtight container for up to three days.

NUTRITION per serving	**34** cals | **2** g protein
	2 g fat (**<1** g saturates)
	1 g carbs (**1** g total sugars)
	2 g fibre

Lemon blueberry cake

· · · · · · · · · · · ·

This healthy, summery cake is perfect for celebrations. Made with rapeseed oil, it is lower in saturated fat and higher in vitamin E than traditional recipes. Here, I have replaced some of the flour with ground almonds, which add fibre, calcium and iron. Blueberries are rich in polyphenols, which promote speedy recovery and reduce inflammation, although you can swap for raspberries or blackberries, which are also rich sources. Baking powder and bicarbonate replace eggs and help create a light, airy texture.

MAKES 10 SLICES

120 ml rapeseed oil
140 g sugar
125 g self-raising flour
100 g ground almonds
2 tsp baking powder
½ tsp bicarbonate of soda
¼ tsp salt
Zest of 2 lemons
50 ml plain plant yogurt
  alternative
100 g blueberries, tossed in flour

TO DECORATE

100 g icing sugar mixed with
  1 tbsp lemon juice
100 g blueberries

Preheat the oven to 160°C/fan 140°C/gas mark 3. Line a 20 cm round cake tin with baking paper.

In a bowl or food mixer, mix together the oil and sugar. Add the flour, almonds, baking powder, bicarbonate of soda, salt, lemon zest and yogurt alternative; mix until combined. Fold in the blueberries (tossing them in flour first helps prevent from them sinking during baking).

Spoon the mixture into the prepared tin, smooth the surface with a knife and bake in the preheated oven for 55–60 minutes until light golden and springy to the touch and a skewer inserted in the centre comes out clean. Leave to cool in the tin for 10 minutes, then turn out onto a wire rack to cool completely.

Make the glacé icing by mixing together the icing sugar and lemon juice in a bowl, then spread over the cooled cake with a knife and top with fresh blueberries.

NUTRITION per slice | **294** cals | **4** g protein | **15** g fat (**1** g saturates) | **36** g carbs (**26** g total sugars) | **2** g fibre

Hummus – three ways

. . . .

Hummus is made from chickpeas, which are brilliant sources of protein, iron and fructo-oligosaccharides, a type of fibre that feeds the friendly bacteria of the gut and benefits the immune system. To make your own, you will need a food processor, then simply blend together chickpeas with the other ingredients. They come together to make a beautifully creamy dip for crunchy vegetables or homemade tortilla crisps (p. 100). Hummus is also delicious on toast, as a topping for baked potatoes or with a salad.

Chickpea hummus

This basic recipe takes minutes to make, is lower in fat than most shop-bought varieties, and tastes far nicer too!

MAKES 350g

400 g can chickpeas, drained
  and rinsed
1 garlic clove, crushed
2 tbsp olive or rapeseed oil
1 tbsp tahini
Juice of ½ lemon
2–4 tbsp water
Salt and freshly ground black
  pepper, to taste

Place all the ingredients in a food processor or blender and blend until smooth. Taste to check the seasoning, then spoon into a shallow dish. It will keep, covered, in the fridge for up to three days. Serve topped with chilli flakes.

NUTRITION
per 1 tablespoon (30 g):
56 cals | **2** g protein
4 g fat (**1** g saturates)
4 g carbs (**<1** g total sugars)
1 g fibre

Carrot, ginger and turmeric hummus

This warming hummus is loaded with immune-supporting antioxidant nutrients, perfect as a dip or with roasted vegetables.

MAKES 525g

400 g can chickpeas, drained
  and rinsed
200 g cooked carrots
2 tbsp olive or rapeseed oil
1 tbsp tahini
1 garlic clove, crushed
Freshly squeezed juice of ½ lemon
1 tsp grated fresh root ginger
¼ tsp turmeric
A pinch of cayenne pepper
2–4 tbsp water
Salt, to taste

Place all the ingredients in the bowl of a food processor and blend for 30 seconds until smooth, then transfer to a bowl. It will keep, covered, in the fridge for up to three days. Serve topped with chopped parsley.

NUTRITION
per 1 tablespoon (30 g):
38 cals | **1** g protein
2 g fat (**<1** g saturates)
3 g carbs (**1** g total sugars)
1 g fibre

Beetroot and horseradish hummus

This vibrant hummus is delicious with salad or spread on toast.

MAKES 500g

400 g can chickpeas, drained
  and rinsed
150 g cooked beetroot
1 garlic clove, crushed
2 tbsp olive or rapeseed oil
1 tbsp tahini
Juice of ½ lemon
½ tsp horseradish sauce
2–4 tbsp water
Salt, to taste
A handful of fresh mint

Place the chickpeas, beetroot, garlic, oil, tahini, lemon juice, horseradish sauce, water and salt in the bowl of a food processor and blend for 30 seconds until smooth. Add the mint, pulse briefly, then transfer to a bowl. It will keep, covered, in the fridge for up to three days. Serve topped with mint leaves.

NUTRITION
per 1 tablespoon (30 g):
43 cals | **2** g protein
2 g fat (**<1** g saturates)
3 g carbs (**<1** g total sugars)
1 g fibre

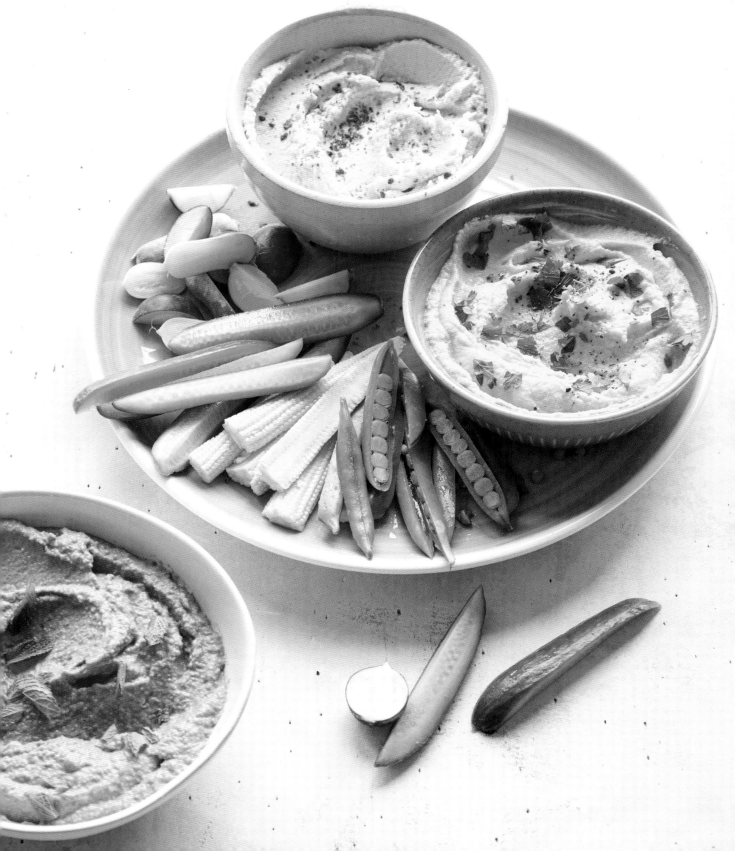

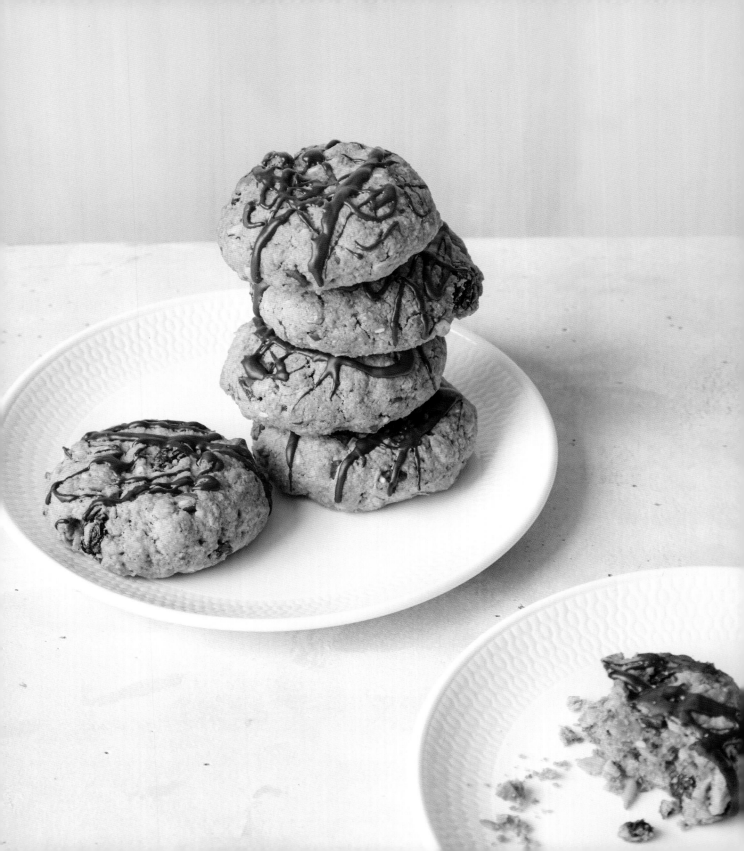

Jumbo oat cookies

· · · · · · · · · · · · ·

These cookies (dubbed Happiness Cookies in my house) are the result of dozens of experiments to create the perfect vegan oat cookie that tastes amazing *and* delivers maximum nutrition. They are packed with chunky oats, nuts, seeds and raisins, which means they deliver plenty of protein, fibre, B vitamins, iron and healthy fat. The secret ingredient that makes them chewy and crisp is golden syrup. It is such an adaptable recipe – you can swap the raisins for any other dried fruit, the almonds for walnuts or use any other nut butter you prefer.

MAKES 16 COOKIES

100 g dairy-free spread
100 g light brown sugar
100 g peanut butter
25 g golden syrup
100 g jumbo oats
50 g ground almonds
100 g wholemeal spelt or
   plain flour
1 tsp cinnamon
2 tbsp plant milk alternative
50 g raisins
50 g dark chocolate chips
25 g mixed seeds

FOR THE TOPPING (OPTIONAL)

25 g plain chocolate, melted

Preheat the oven to 180°C/fan 160°C/gas mark 4. Meanwhile, line two baking sheets with baking paper.

Mix together the dairy-free spread and sugar in a bowl, then add the nut butter and golden syrup.

In a large bowl, mix together the oats, ground almonds, flour and cinnamon, then add the dry ingredients to the wet ingredients, mixing until just combined. Stir in the plant milk alternative. You should now have a fairly stiff mixture that's sticky enough to be rolled into a ball. If it's too crumbly, add extra milk. Add the raisins, chocolate chips and seeds and mix in.

Form the mixture into 16 balls, place on the prepared baking sheets and flatten them slightly. Bake for approximately 15 minutes – the edges should be firm and the tops golden. Leave to cool for a few minutes before transferring to a wire rack to cool completely. When cool, drizzle with melted chocolate, if liked. These will keep for up to a week in an airtight container.

NUTRITION per cookie* | **202** cals | **5** g protein | **11** g fat (**2** g saturates) | **21** g carbs (**12** g total sugars) | **2** g fibre

*without topping

Peanut butter bars

· · · · · · · · · · · · · ·

These super-nutritious no bake bars are ideal post-workout snacks. Equally, they can be consumed anytime you want a tasty energy boost. They combine crunchy seeds, nuts and oats with peanut butter, so they are loaded with protein, healthy fat, B vitamins, iron, zinc and magnesium. You can substitute any other type of nut butter for peanut butter if you wish. Healthy refuelling never tasted so good!

MAKES 12 BARS

25 g pumpkin seeds
50 g flaked almonds
25 g desiccated coconut
25 g sesame seeds
125 g rolled oats
50 g raisins
50 g dark chocolate chips
85 ml maple syrup
200 g peanut butter
1 tsp vanilla extract

Line a 18 cm square tin with baking paper. Meanwhile, toast the pumpkin seeds, almonds, coconut and sesame seeds under a hot grill for 2–3 minutes or until lightly golden. Allow to cool. Add them to a large mixing bowl with the oats, raisins and chocolate chips and mix together well.

Place the maple syrup, peanut butter and vanilla extract in a small saucepan and heat gently until melted. Combine the liquid mixture with the dry ingredients until all dry ingredients are coated. Press evenly into the tin and refrigerate for at least 2–3 hours before slicing into bars.

NUTRITION per bar | **266** cals | **9** g protein | **17** g fat (**4** g saturates) | **19** g carbs (**10** g total sugars) | **4** g fibre

Three-nut butter

....

With so many varieties of nut and seed butters available from supermarkets, you may wonder why you should bother making your own. Well, for a start, homemade nut butter tastes far nicer than anything you can buy from a shop – and it's fun to experiment with different types and flavour combinations. This recipe uses three different types of nut, which gives you plenty of omega-3s, plus a touch of maple syrup, which helps the mixture emulsify (blend together). You can, of course, substitute any other nut combination you fancy or just use one type of nut or seed, such as peanuts, cashews, pumpkin seeds, pistachios or sunflower seeds. Whichever variety you choose, all nuts and seeds are brilliant sources of healthy fats, protein, fibre, B vitamins, iron, zinc and magnesium. It is well worth the effort of toasting the nuts first as this enhances the flavour of the nut butter. A high-speed food processor or blender gives the smoothest results.

MAKES
APPROXIMATELY 300g

100 g walnuts
100 g pecans
100 g almonds
A pinch of salt
1 tbsp maple syrup

Preheat the oven to 180°C/fan 160°C/gas mark 4.

Spread the nuts in an even layer on a baking tray and place in the oven for 8–10 minutes. Check them often (they have a tendency to burn easily) and shake the tray halfway through the cooking time to make sure all the nuts are toasting evenly.

Place the toasted nuts in the bowl of a high-speed food processor or blender along with the salt and maple syrup; blend until a creamy butter forms. This can take 10–12 minutes, so be patient – it is worth the wait! It's a good idea to let the machine pause every few minutes to avoid straining it. You may also need to scrape down the sides of the blender with a spatula a couple of times.

Transfer the mixture to a clean glass jar and cover it. The nut butter will keep in the fridge for up to three weeks, but is best consumed at room temperature.

NUTRITION per 15 g (level tablespoon) | **101** cals | **3** g protein | **9** g fat (**1** g saturates) | **1** g carbs (**1** g total sugars) | **1** g fibre

Protein balls

....

As well as being high in protein, these tasty balls also deliver generous amounts of vitamin E, magnesium and zinc to aid your recovery after a training session. You can substitute almond or cashew butter for the peanut butter, or raisins or mixed seeds for the chocolate chips. It takes just 10 minutes to whip up a batch and they can be stored in the fridge for up to a week.

MAKES 24 BALLS

125 g rolled oats
250 g peanut butter
75 g golden, agave or maple syrup
2 scoops (50 g) chocolate vegan
   protein powder
2 tbsp plain chocolate chips

Place all the ingredients in the bowl of a food processor and blitz until a stiff 'dough' forms, adding a little water if the mixture seems too crumbly. Alternatively, stir together in a mixing bowl – you may need to use your hands to knead the dough near the end.

Form the dough into 24 balls. Transfer to an airtight container and store in the fridge for up to a week, or in the freezer for up to three months.

NUTRITION per ball | **111** cals | **5** g protein | **6** g fat (**1** g saturates) | **8** g carbs (**4** g total sugars) | **1** g fibre

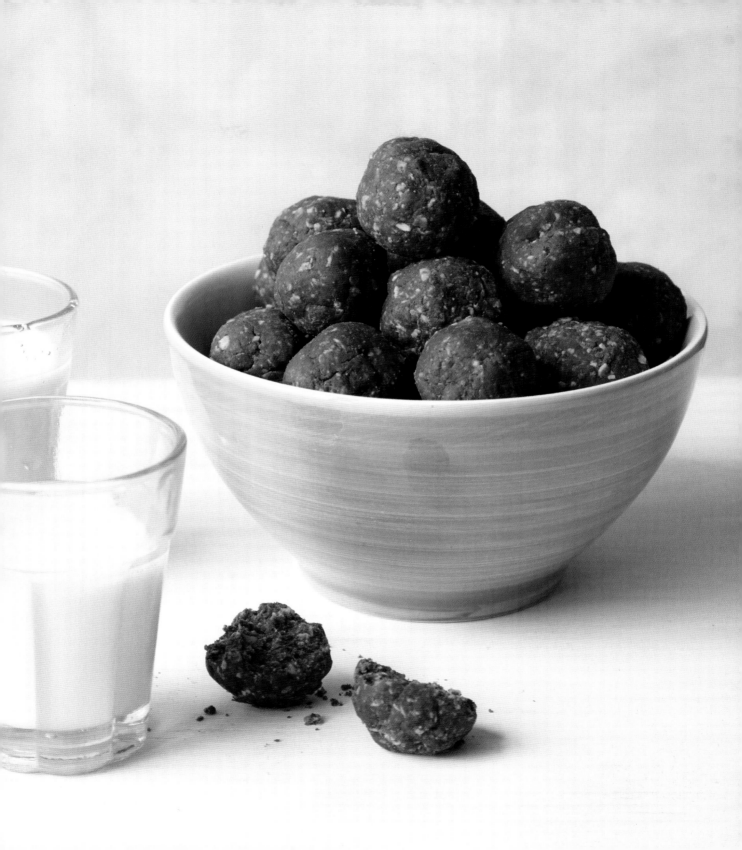

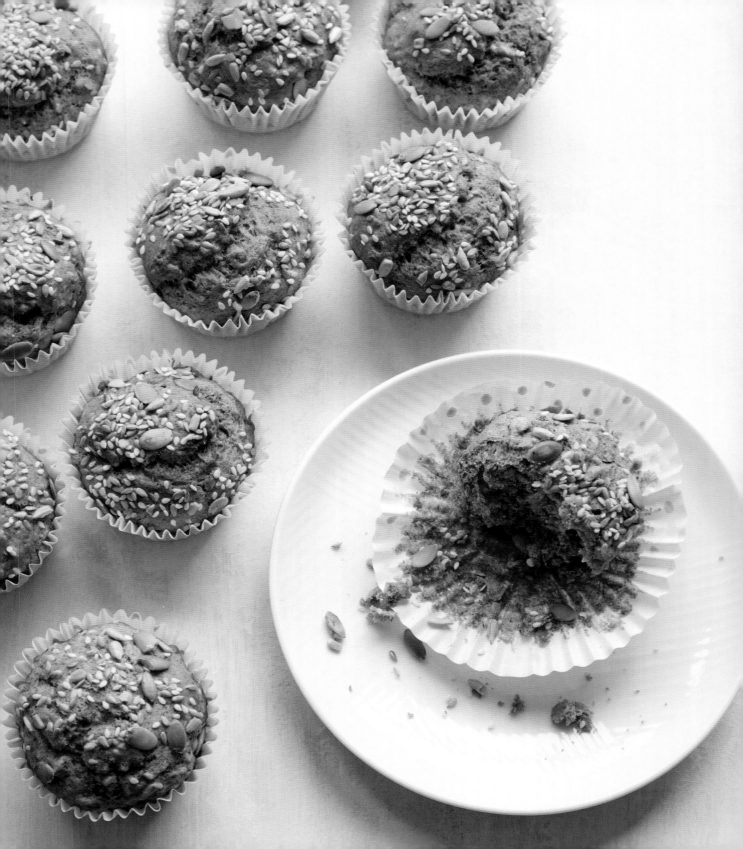

Seeded banana muffins

. . . .

These tasty muffins are ideal for popping in your kit bag or lunchbox for fuelling on the go. Made with mixed seeds and olive oil, they are loaded with healthy omega-3 fats, fibre and zinc. They contain less saturated fat and sugar than traditional banana cake and are guaranteed to provide you with long-lasting energy. A batch of these should keep for a couple of days in an airtight container, although they don't last long in my house! Alternatively, I recommend wrapping individually in foil and freezing so you can just take out and defrost as needed.

MAKES 12 MUFFINS

200 g self-raising flour
1 tsp baking powder
½ tsp bicarbonate of soda
1½ tsp ground cinnamon
3 ripe bananas, peeled
50 g light brown sugar
50 ml maple syrup
50 ml light olive or rapeseed oil
1½ tsp vanilla extract
75 g mixed seeds, plus 1 tbsp
   extra for topping (or any
   mixture of sunflower seeds,
   pumpkin seeds, sesame
   seeds and linseeds)

Preheat the oven to 200°C/fan 180°C/gas mark 6. Meanwhile, line 12 muffin tins with paper cases.

Mix the flour, baking powder, bicarbonate of soda and cinnamon in a large mixing bowl. In a separate bowl, mash the bananas, sugar and maple syrup, then mix in the oil and vanilla. Add to the flour. Stir until just combined, then mix in the seeds.

Divide the mixture among the muffin cases, sprinkle over the extra seeds and bake for approximately 20 minutes until the muffins are risen and golden. Leave to cool for 10 minutes in the muffin tin before removing and leave to cool completely on a wire rack.

NUTRITION per muffin | **180** cals | **4** g protein | **7** g fat (**1** g saturates) | **25** g carbs (**11** g total sugars) | **2** g fibre

Super-seedy bars

. . . .

I wanted to create a snack bar that delivered maximum possible nutrition plus fantastic taste and here is the result: super-seedy, crunchy, nutty, heavenly bars that are high in fibre, omega-3 fats, protein, B vitamins, vitamin E, magnesium, iron and zinc. Nuts and seeds are real powerhouses of nutrients and therefore form the basis of these bars. They team beautifully with dark chocolate, which packs a hefty polyphenol punch. Perfect after exercise or anytime you want a nutritious treat.

MAKES 8

125 g mixed seeds (or any combination of sunflower, pumpkin, sesame and flaxseeds)
100 g mixed nuts (or any combination of almonds, cashews, Brazil nuts and pecans), roughly chopped
25 g ground flaxseed
25 g rolled oats
1 tsp vanilla extract
½ tsp cinnamon
75 ml golden, agave or maple syrup
50 g dark chocolate (at least 70 per cent cocoa)

Preheat the oven to 180°C/fan 160°C/gas mark 4. Meanwhile, line a 900 g loaf tin (18 x 6 cm) with baking paper.

Place the seeds, nuts, flaxseed and oats in a large mixing bowl. Add the vanilla extract, cinnamon and syrup; mix together. Spoon into the prepared tin. Press down firmly, making sure there are no gaps, and bake for about 30 minutes until lightly golden but not brown around the edges. Take out of the oven and press down again using a large spoon. Allow to cool completely.

Break the chocolate into small pieces, place in a microwavable bowl and heat on full power for 2–3 minutes, stirring at 30-second intervals until almost molten. Stir and leave for a few moments until completely melted. Alternatively, place the chocolate pieces in a heatproof bowl set over a pan of gently simmering water, and heat until the chocolate starts to melt, then stir until completely melted. Drizzle over the cooled nut mixture. Pop the tin in the freezer for the chocolate to set, otherwise you can just leave to cool in the kitchen. Once cooled, cut into eight bars. They will keep in an airtight container for up to seven days.

NUTRITION per bar | **266** cals | **8** g protein | **18** g fat (**4** g saturates) | **16** g carbs (**12** g total sugars) | **4** g fibre

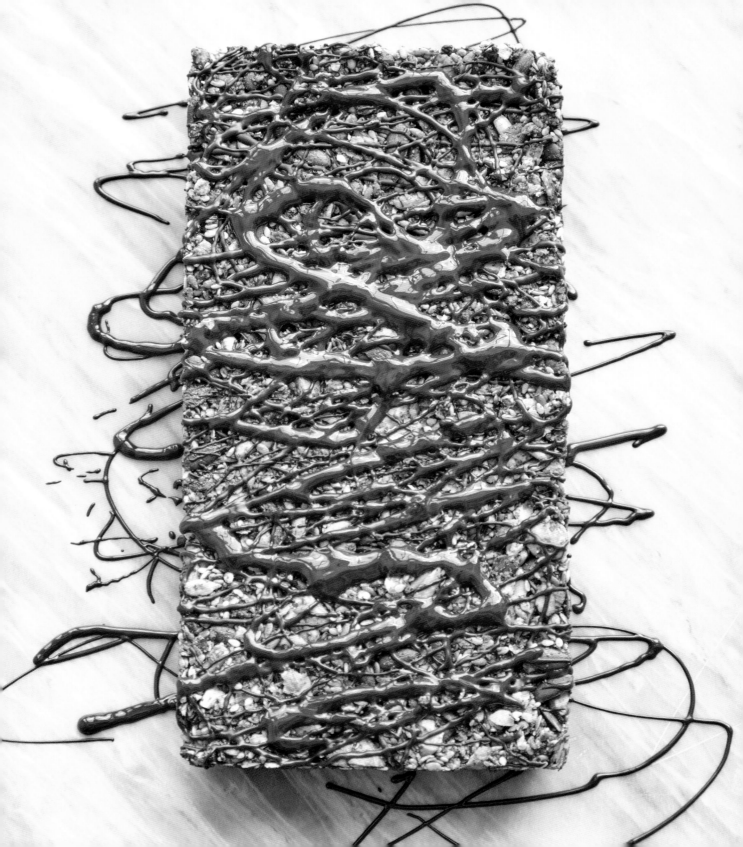

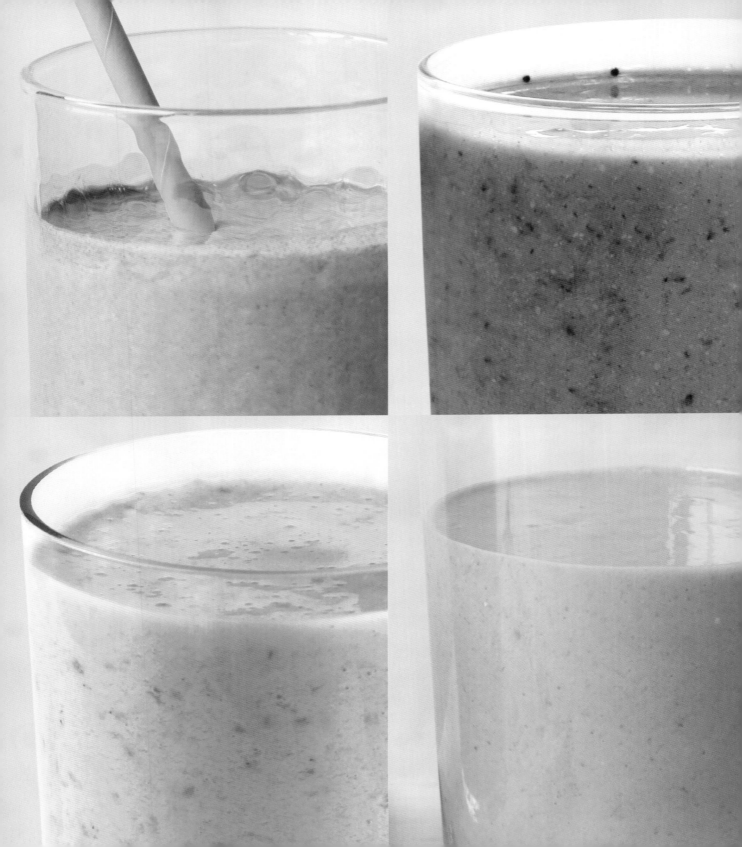

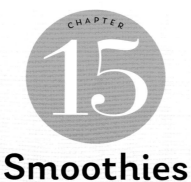

15

Smoothies

Power-up cinnamon coffee smoothie

············

This energising smoothie is perfect before a workout when you don't have time for a balanced meal. It gives you the performance-enhancing benefits of caffeine and the energy-boosting benefits of bananas, so will help keep you fuelled and alert. Two shots of espresso provide around 150 mg caffeine, which studies show can increase stamina and reduce the perception of effort.

SERVES 1

200 ml almond milk alternative
1–2 shots (50–100 ml) espresso
1 tbsp almond butter
1 banana, peeled and chopped
1 tsp cinnamon
Agave or maple syrup, to taste
A few ice cubes

Place all the ingredients in a blender or food processor and blend until smooth. Pour into a tall glass.

NUTRITION per serving	206 cals | **6** g protein
	11 g fat (**1** g saturates)
	20 g carbs (**18** g total sugars)
	4 g fibre

Strawberry cashew smoothie

············

This delicious smoothie is packed with protein and antioxidant nutrients, making it the perfect post-workout option. It delivers 25 g protein, the ideal amount for promoting muscle building and repair after exercise. Cashews provide a boost of healthy fats and fibre, while strawberries are loaded with vitamin C, delivering your entire daily requirement.

SERVES 1

25 g cashew nuts
250 ml plant milk alternative (any type)
100 g strawberries, fresh or frozen
2 tsp lemon juice
1 scoop (25 g) vanilla vegan protein powder
A few ice cubes (optional)

Place all the ingredients in a blender or food processor and blend until smooth (adding a few ice cubes if you want a thicker smoothie). Pour into a tall glass.

NUTRITION per serving	307 cals | **25** g protein
	16 g fat (**3** g saturates)
	14 g carbs (**7** g total sugars)
	6 g fibre

Mixed berry chia smoothie

············

This delicious smoothie makes an ideal recovery drink, providing 25 g protein and a rich source of polyphenols, which help reduce oxidative stress and inflammation, and improve blood vessel function and blood flow. It also contains chia seeds, one tablespoon of which provides your entire daily requirement for omega-3s. They also give the smoothie more texture, with a little bit of crunch. I prefer making this smoothie with almond milk alternative, but you can use any other type.

SERVES 1

125 ml plain yogurt alternative
   (soya, almond or coconut)
125 ml almond milk alternative
100 g frozen mixed berries
Juice of ½ lime
½ scoop (15 g) vanilla vegan
   protein powder
1 tbsp nut butter (any type)
1 tbsp chia seeds

Place all the ingredients in a blender or food processor, reserving a few berries for decoration, and blend until smooth. Add a little water for a thinner consistency or extra nut butter for creaminess and top with the remaining berries.

NUTRITION
per serving | 337 cals | **25** g protein | **17** g fat (**3** g saturates) | **17** g carbs (**4** g total sugars) | **11** g fibre

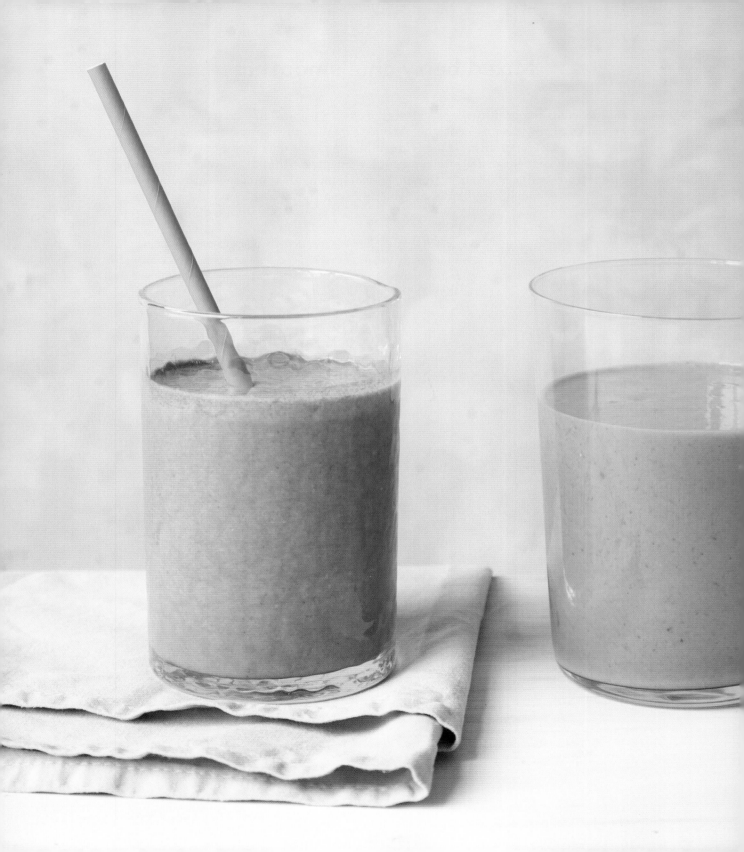

Protein oat smoothie

....

Smoothies make a very healthy breakfast and are the perfect solution when you are pressed for time. This high-protein recipe, with oats, nut butter and banana, is both filling and nutritious. Oats are rich in fibre and they make the smoothie satisfyingly thick so you will feel full all morning. Frozen bananas make the smoothie thick and creamy – simply peel, cut into pieces, then freeze them in a zip-top bag. If you do not have any frozen bananas, you can use fresh banana and add a few ice cubes at the end to thicken it up. Ground flaxseed is rich in omega-3s, while the nut butter also makes this smoothie nutritious and filling. Strawberries provide plenty of vitamin C, but any other berries will work equally well.

SERVES 1

25 g rolled oats
250 ml almond milk alternative (or any other type)
½ scoop (15 g) vanilla or chocolate vegan protein powder
½ banana, peeled, chopped into chunks and frozen
60 g frozen strawberries (or other berries)
1 tbsp ground flaxseed
1 tbsp nut butter
Ice (optional)

Place the oats in a blender or food processor and pulse until finely ground. Add the remaining ingredients and blend until smooth. If you want a thicker smoothie, add ice. That's it!

NUTRITION per serving	**421** cals | **24** g protein
	19 g fat (**3** g saturates)
	35 g carbs (**14** g total sugars)
	10 g fibre

Mango green protein smoothie

....

This healthy green smoothie with spinach, mango and banana tastes like a tropical holiday! It is a brilliant way to get an extra serving of green veg into your diet – spinach is an excellent source of vitamin K, beta-carotene, folate and vitamin C, plus iron and magnesium. When combined with mango, you cannot taste it. Mango is packed with beta-carotene and vitamin C, while bananas deliver potassium and fibre. You can swap the banana for fresh or canned pineapple chunks if you prefer.

SERVES 1

1 scoop (25 g) vanilla vegan protein powder
250 ml plant milk alternative
2 handfuls (about 50 g) baby spinach
200 g frozen mango pieces
1 banana, peeled and sliced

Place all the ingredients in a blender or food processor and blend until smooth. Add a little water or extra plant milk alternative if you want a thinner consistency, then pour into a tall glass.

NUTRITION per serving	**346** cals | **23** g protein
	4 g fat (**1** g saturates)
	50 g carbs (**44** g total sugars)
	10 g fibre

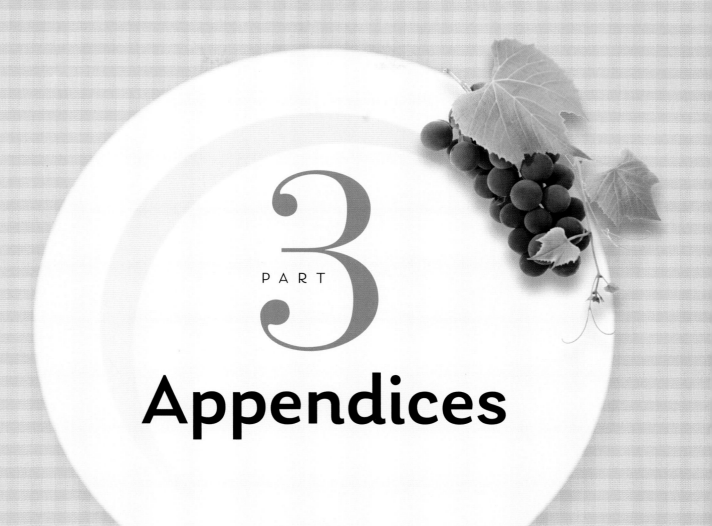

PART

3

Appendices

Acknowledgements

This book has been a dream of mine for a long time and would not have been possible without the help of many talented people.

Thank you to my wonderful team at Bloomsbury for their vision and support: publisher Charlotte Croft, senior editor Holly Jarrald, copy editor Jane Donovan, proof-reader Nicky Gyopari, designer Austin Taylor, cover designer James Watson, head of marketing Lizzy Ewer, senior publicity manager Katherine MacPherson and senior marketing executive Alice Graham. It has been an absolute privilege to work with you.

The stunning photographs in this book are thanks to photographer Clare Winfield and food stylist Emily Kydd. You have done an outstanding job.

I am also very grateful to Liz Smith and Gill McPherson for their help with testing the recipes.

And, lastly, a huge thank you to my incredible husband, Simon, who is my rock, and my beautiful daughters, Chloe and Lucy, who provide me with motivation for everything I do.

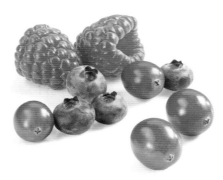

References

Introduction

1   **The Vegan Society.** 'Statistics', https://www.vegansociety.com/news/media/statistics. Accessed September 2020.

2   **The Waitrose Food & Drink Report 2018–2019.** https://www.waitrose.com/content/dam/waitrose/Inspiration/About%20Us%20New/Food%20and%20drink%20report%202017/foodanddrinkreport1920v2.pdf. Accessed September 2020.

3   **The Vegetarian Resource Group (VRG).** 'How Many Adults in the U.S. Are Vegetarian and Vegan', https://www.vrg.org/nutshell/Polls/2016_adults_veg.htm. Accessed September 2020.

4   **Friends of the Earth Europe.** 'Meat Atlas', https://www.foeeurope.org/sites/default/files/publications/foee_hbf_meatatlas_jan2014.pdf. Accessed September 2020.

Chapter 1

1   **Mariotti, François, Gardner, Christopher D.** 'Dietary Protein and Amino Acids in Vegetarian Diets—A Review', *Nutrients*, vol. 11, no. 11, November 2019, p. 2661. *www.mdpi.com*, doi:10.3390/nu11112661.

2   **Sobiecki, Jakub G, et al.** 'High Compliance with Dietary Recommendations in a Cohort of Meat Eaters, Fish Eaters, Vegetarians, and Vegans: Results from the European Prospective Investigation into Cancer and Nutrition-Oxford Study', Nutrition Research (New York, N.Y.), vol. 36, no. 5, May 2016, pp. 464–77. PubMed, doi:10.1016/j.nutres.2015.12.016.

3   **Melina, Vesanto, et al.** 'Position of the Academy of Nutrition and Dietetics: Vegetarian Diets', *Journal of the Academy of Nutrition and Dietetics*, vol. 116, no. 12, December 2016, pp. 1970–80. *jandonline.org*, doi:10.1016/j.jand.2016.09.025.

4   **BDA.** *Plant-Based Diet*, https://www.bda.uk.com/resource/plant-based-diet.html. Accessed September 2020.

5   **Morton, Robert W, et al.** 'A Systematic Review, Meta-Analysis and Meta-Regression of the Effect of Protein Supplementation on Resistance Training-Induced Gains in Muscle Mass and Strength in Healthy Adults', *British Journal of Sports Medicine*, vol. 52, no. 6, March 2018, pp. 376–84. *bjsm.bmj.com*, doi:10.1136/bjsports-2017-097608.

6   **Messina, Mark, et al.** 'No Difference Between the Effects of Supplementing With Soy Protein Versus Animal Protein on Gains in Muscle Mass and Strength in Response to Resistance Exercise', *International Journal of Sport Nutrition and Exercise Metabolism*, vol. 28, no. 6, November 2018, pp. 674–85. *journals.humankinetics.com*, doi:10.1123/ijsnem.2018-0071.

7   **Moore, Daniel R, et al.** 'Ingested Protein Dose Response of Muscle and Albumin Protein Synthesis after Resistance Exercise in Young Men', *The American Journal of Clinical Nutrition*, vol. 89, no. 1, January 2009, pp. 161–68. *PubMed*, doi:10.3945/ajcn.2008.26401.

8   **McDougall, John.** 'Plant Foods Have a Complete Amino Acid Composition', *Circulation*, vol. 105, no. 25, June 2002, pp. e197–e197. *ahajournals.org (Atypon)*, doi:10.1161/01.CIR.0000018905.97677.1F.

9   **Gardner, Christopher D, et al.** 'Maximizing the Intersection of Human Health and the Health of the Environment with Regard to the Amount and Type of Protein Produced and Consumed in the United States', *Nutrition Reviews*, vol. 77, no. 4, April 2019, pp. 197–215. *academic.oup.com*, doi:10.1093/nutrit/nuy073.

10 **Lappé, Frances Moore, Marika Hahn.** *Diet for a Small Planet*, Ballantine Books, 2010. *Open WorldCat.*

11 **Young, V R, and Pellett, P L.** 'Plant Proteins in Relation to Human Protein and Amino Acid Nutrition', *The American Journal of Clinical Nutrition*, vol. 59, no. 5 Suppl, 1994, pp. 1203S–1212S. *PubMed*, doi:10.1093/ajcn/59.5.1203S.

12 **Craddock, J C, et al.** 'Plant-based Eating Patterns and Endurance Performance: A Focus on Inflammation, Oxidative Stress and Immune Responses', *Nutrition Bulletin*, vol. 45, no. 2, June 2020, pp. 123–32. *DOI.org (Crossref)*, doi:10.1111/nbu.12427.

13 **Li, Ni, et al.** 'Soy and Isoflavone Consumption and Multiple Health Outcomes: Umbrella Review of Systematic Reviews and Meta-Analyses of Observational Studies and Randomized Trials in Humans', *Molecular Nutrition & Food Research*, vol. 64, no. 4, 2020, p. 1900751. *Wiley Online Library*, doi:10.1002/mnfr.201900751.

14 **Rizzo, Gianluca, Baroni, Luciana.** 'Soy, Soy Foods and Their Role in Vegetarian Diets', *Nutrients*, vol. 10, no. 1, January 2018. PubMed Central, doi:10.3390/nu10010043.

15 **Chen, Meinan, et al.** 'Association between Soy Isoflavone Intake and Breast Cancer Risk for Pre- and Post-Menopausal Women: A Meta-Analysis of Epidemiological Studies', *PLOS One*, vol. 9, no. 2, 2014, p. e89288. PubMed, doi:10.1371/journal.pone.0089288.

16 **Lee, Sang-Ah, et al.** 'Adolescent and Adult Soy Food Intake and Breast Cancer Risk: Results from the Shanghai Women's Health Study', *The American Journal of Clinical Nutrition*, vol. 89, no. 6, June 2009, pp. 1920–26. PubMed, doi:10.3945/ajcn.2008.27361.

Chapter 2

1 **Medawar, Evelyn, et al.** 'The Effects of Plant-Based Diets on the Body and the Brain: A Systematic Review', *Translational Psychiatry*, vol. 9, no. 1, September 2019, pp. 1–17. www.nature.com, doi:10.1038/s41398-019-0552-0.

2 **Melina, Vesanto, et al.** 'Position of the Academy of Nutrition and Dietetics: Vegetarian Diets', *Journal of the Academy of Nutrition and Dietetics*, vol. 116, no. 12, 2016, pp. 1970–80. PubMed, doi:10.1016/j.jand.2016.09.025.

3 **BDA.** 'Plant-Based Diet', https://www.bda.uk.com/resource/plant-based-diet.html. Accessed September 2020.

4 **Kim, Hyunju, et al.** 'Healthy Plant-Based Diets Are Associated with Lower Risk of All-Cause Mortality in US Adults', *The Journal of Nutrition*, vol. 148, no. 4, 01 2018, pp. 624–31. PubMed, doi:10.1093/jn/nxy019.

5 **Lassale, Camille, et al.** 'Abstract 16: A Pro-Vegetarian Food Pattern and Cardiovascular Mortality in the Epic Study', *Circulation*, vol. 131, no. suppl_1 March 2015, pp. A16–A16. ahajournals.org (Atypon), doi:10.1161/circ.131.suppl_1.16.

6 **Phillips, R L, et al.** 'Coronary Heart Disease Mortality among Seventh-Day Adventists with Differing Dietary Habits: A Preliminary Report', *The American Journal of Clinical Nutrition*, vol. 31, no. 10 Suppl, 1978, pp. S191–98. PubMed, doi:10.1093/ajcn/31.10.S191.

7 **Singh, Pramil N, et al.** 'Does Low Meat Consumption Increase Life Expectancy in Humans?' *The American Journal of Clinical Nutrition*, vol. 78, no. 3, September 2003, pp. 526S–532S. academic.oup.com, doi:10.1093/ajcn/78.3.526S.

8 **Thomas, D Travis, et al.** 'American College of Sports Medicine Joint Position Statement. Nutrition and Athletic Performance', *Medicine and Science in Sports and Exercise*, vol. 48, no. 3, March 2016, pp. 543–68. PubMed, doi:10.1249/MSS.0000000000000852.

9 **Le, Lap Tai, Sabaté, Joan.** 'Beyond Meatless, the Health Effects of Vegan Diets: Findings from the Adventist Cohorts', *Nutrients*, vol. 6, no. 6, May 2014, pp. 2131–47. PubMed Central, doi:10.3390/nu6062131.

10 **Key, Timothy J, et al.** 'Mortality in Vegetarians and Nonvegetarians: Detailed Findings from a Collaborative

Analysis of 5 Prospective Studies', *The American Journal of Clinical Nutrition*, vol. 70, no. 3, September 1999, pp. 516s–24s. academic.oup.com, doi:10.1093/ajcn/70.3.516s.

11 **Aykan, Nuri Faruk.** 'Red Meat and Colorectal Cancer', *Oncology Reviews*, vol. 9, no. 1, December 2015. PubMed Central, doi:10.4081/oncol.2015.288.

12 **Afshin, Ashkan, et al.** 'Health Effects of Dietary Risks in 195 Countries, 1990–2017: A Systematic Analysis for the Global Burden of Disease Study 2017', *The Lancet*, vol. 393, no. 10184, May 2019, pp. 1958–72. www.thelancet.com, doi:10.1016/S0140-6736(19)30041-8.

13 **Budhathoki, Sanjeev, et al.** 'Association of Animal and Plant Protein Intake With All-Cause and Cause-Specific Mortality in a Japanese Cohort', *JAMA Internal Medicine*, vol. 179, no. 11, November 2019, pp. 1509–18. jamanetwork.com, doi:10.1001/jamainternmed.2019.2806.

14 **Ahnen, Rylee T, et al.** 'Role of Plant Protein in Nutrition, Wellness, and Health', *Nutrition Reviews*, vol. 77, no. 11, November 2019, pp. 735–47. academic.oup.com, doi:10.1093/nutrit/nuz028.

15 **Hosseinpour-Niazi, S, et al.** 'Substitution of Red Meat with Legumes in the Therapeutic Lifestyle Change Diet Based on Dietary Advice Improves Cardiometabolic Risk Factors in Overweight Type 2 Diabetes Patients: A Cross-over Randomized Clinical Trial', *European Journal of Clinical Nutrition*, vol. 69, no. 5, May 2015, pp. 592–97. PubMed, doi:10.1038/ejcn.2014.228.

16 **Dinu, Monica, et al.** 'Vegetarian, Vegan Diets and Multiple Health Outcomes: A Systematic Review with Meta-Analysis of Observational Studies', *Critical Reviews in Food Science and Nutrition*, vol. 57, no. 17, November 2017, pp. 3640–49. PubMed, doi:10.1080/10408398.2016.1138447.

17 **Crowe, Francesca L, et al.** 'Risk of Hospitalization or Death from Ischemic Heart Disease among British Vegetarians and Nonvegetarians: Results from the EPIC-Oxford Cohort Study', *The American Journal of Clinical Nutrition*, vol. 97, no. 3, March 2013, pp. 597–603. PubMed, doi:10.3945/ajcn.112.044073.

18 **Chang-Claude, J, Frentzel-Beyme, R.** 'Dietary and Lifestyle Determinants of Mortality among German Vegetarians', *International Journal of Epidemiology*, vol. 22, no. 2, April 1993, pp. 228–36. PubMed, doi:10.1093/ije/22.2.228.

19 **World Cancer Research Fund.** 'Diet, Nutrition, Physical Activity and Cancer: A Global Perspective The Third Expert Report', 2018.

20 **Thomas, D Travis, et al.** 'American College of Sports Medicine Joint Position Statement. Nutrition and Athletic Performance', *Medicine and Science in Sports and Exercise*, vol. 48, no. 3, March 2016, pp. 543–68. PubMed, doi:10.1249/MSS.0000000000000852.

21 **Longo, Umile Giuseppe, et al.** 'The Best Athletes in Ancient Rome Were Vegetarian!', *Journal of Sports Science & Medicine*, vol. 7, no. 4, December 2008, p. 565.

22 **Barr, Susan I, Rideout, Candice A.** 'Nutritional Considerations for Vegetarian Athletes', *Nutrition* (Burbank, Los Angeles County, Calif.), vol. 20, no. 7–8, August 2004, pp. 696–703. PubMed, doi:10.1016/j.nut.2004.04.015.

23 **Eisinger, M.** 'Nutrient intake of endurance runners with lacto-ovo vegetarian diet and regular Western diet'. *Z. Ernahrungswiss*, vol. 33, 1994, pp. 217–29.

24 **Craddock, Joel C, et al.** 'Vegetarian and Omnivorous Nutrition – Comparing Physical Performance', *International Journal of Sport Nutrition and Exercise Metabolism*, vol. 26, no. 3, June 2016, pp. 212–20. PubMed, doi:10.1123/ijsnem.2015-0231.

25 **Lynch, Heidi M, et al.** 'Cardiorespiratory Fitness and Peak Torque Differences between Vegetarian and Omnivore Endurance Athletes: A Cross-Sectional Study', *Nutrients*, vol. 8, no. 11, November 2016, p. 726. www.mdpi.com, doi:10.3390/nu8110726.

26 **Nebl, Josefine, et al.** 'Exercise Capacity of Vegan, Lacto-Ovo-Vegetarian and Omnivorous Recreational Runners', *Journal of the International Society of Sports Nutrition*, vol. 16, no. 1, May 2019, p. 23. BioMed Central, doi:10.1186/s12970-019-0289-4.

27 **Davey, Gwyneth K, et al.** 'EPIC-Oxford: Lifestyle Characteristics and Nutrient Intakes in a Cohort of 33 883 Meat-Eaters and 31 546 Non Meat-Eaters in the UK', *Public Health Nutrition*, vol. 6, no. 3, May 2003, pp. 259–69. PubMed, doi:10.1079/PHN2002430.

28 **Hughes, Riley L.** 'A Review of the Role of the Gut Microbiome in Personalized Sports Nutrition', *Frontiers in Nutrition*, vol. 6, 2020. Frontiers, doi:10.3389/fnut.2019.00191.

29 **Trapp, Denise, et al.** 'Could a Vegetarian Diet Reduce Exercise-Induced Oxidative Stress? A Review of the Literature', *Journal of Sports Sciences*, vol. 28, no. 12, October 2010, pp. 1261–68. Taylor and Francis+NEJM, doi:10.1080/02640414.2010.507676.

30 **Mach, Núria, Fuster-Botella, Dolors.** 'Endurance Exercise and Gut Microbiota: A Review', *Journal of Sport and Health Science*, vol. 6, no. 2, June 2017, pp. 179–97. PubMed, doi:10.1016/j.jshs.2016.05.001.

31 **Haghighatdoost, Fahimeh, et al.** 'Association of Vegetarian Diet with Inflammatory Biomarkers: A Systematic Review and Meta-Analysis of Observational Studies', *Public Health Nutrition*, vol. 20, no. 15, October 2017, pp. 2713–21. PubMed, doi:10.1017/S1368980017001768.

32 **Igwe, E O, et al.** 'A Systematic Literature Review of the Effect of Anthocyanins on Gut Microbiota Populations', *Journal of Human Nutrition and Dietetics: The Official Journal of the British Dietetic Association*, vol. 32, no. 1, 2019, pp. 53–62. PubMed, doi:10.1111/jhn.12582.

33 **David, Lawrence A, et al.** 'Diet Rapidly and Reproducibly Alters the Human Gut Microbiome', *Nature*, vol. 505, no. 7484, January 2014, pp. 559–63. PubMed, doi:10.1038/nature12820.

34 **McDonald, Daniel, et al.** 'American Gut: An Open Platform for Citizen Science Microbiome Research', *MSystems*, vol. 3, no. 3, June 2018. msystems.asm.org, doi:10.1128/mSystems.00031-18.

35 **Clarke, Siobhan F, et al.** 'Exercise and Associated Dietary Extremes Impact on Gut Microbial Diversity', *Gut*, vol. 63, no. 12, December 2014, pp. 1913–20. PubMed, doi:10.1136/gutjnl-2013-306541.

36 **O'Donovan, Ciara M, et al.** 'Distinct Microbiome Composition and Metabolome Exists across Subgroups of Elite Irish Athletes', *Journal of Science and Medicine in Sport*, vol. 23, no. 1, January 2020, pp. 63–68. www.jsams.org, doi:10.1016/j.jsams.2019.08.290.

37 **Allen, Jacob M, et al.** 'Exercise Alters Gut Microbiota Composition and Function in Lean and Obese Humans', *Medicine and Science in Sports and Exercise*, vol. 50, no. 4, 2018, pp. 747–57. PubMed, doi:10.1249/MSS.0000000000001495.

38 **de Oliveira, Erick Prado, et al.** 'Gastrointestinal Complaints During Exercise: Prevalence, Etiology, and Nutritional Recommendations', *Sports Medicine (Auckland, N.Z.)*, vol. 44, no. Suppl 1, 2014, pp. 79–85. PubMed Central, doi:10.1007/s40279-014-0153-2.

39 **Pugh, Jamie N, et al.** 'Prevalence, Severity and Potential Nutritional Causes of Gastrointestinal Symptoms during a Marathon in Recreational Runners', *Nutrients*, vol. 10, no. 7, June 2018. PubMed, doi:10.3390/nu10070811.

40 **Pugh, Jamie N, et al.** 'Four Weeks of Probiotic Supplementation Reduces GI Symptoms during a Marathon Race', *European Journal of Applied Physiology*, vol. 119, no. 7, July 2019, pp. 1491–501. Springer Link, doi:10.1007/s00421-019-04136-3.

41 **Sranacharoenpong, Kitti, et al.** 'The Environmental Cost of Protein Food Choices', *Public Health Nutrition*, vol. 18, no. 11, August 2015, pp. 2067–73. PubMed, doi:10.1017/S1368980014002377.

42 **Ranganathan, Janet, et al.** 'Shifting Diets for a Sustainable Food Future', April 2016. www.wri.org, https://www.wri.org/publication/shifting-diets.

43 **FAO – News Article: Key Facts and Findings.** http://www.fao.org/news/story/en/item/197623/icode/. Accessed September 2020.

44 **Poore, J, Nemecek, T.** 'Reducing Food's Environmental Impacts through Producers and Consumers', *Science*, vol. 360, no. 6392, June 2018, pp. 987–92. science.sciencemag.org, doi:10.1126/science.aaq0216.

45 **Springmann, Marco, et al.** 'Health and Nutritional Aspects of Sustainable Diet Strategies and Their Association with Environmental Impacts: A Global Modelling Analysis with Country-Level Detail', *The Lancet Planetary Health*, vol. 2, no. 10, October 2018, pp. e451–61. www.thelancet.com, doi:10.1016/S2542-5196(18)30206-7.

46 **Hallström, E, et al.** 'Environmental Impact of Dietary Change: A Systematic Review', *Journal of Cleaner Production*, vol. 91, March 2015, pp. 1–11. ScienceDirect, doi:10.1016/j.jclepro.2014.12.008.

47 **EAT.** 'The EAT-Lancet Commission on Food, Planet, Health – EAT Knowledge', https://eatforum.org/eat-lancet-commission/. Accessed September 2020.

48 **'The Eatwell Guide: A More Sustainable Diet',** https://www.Carbontrust.Com/Resources/the-Eatwell-Guide-a-More-Sustainable-Diet, 21 January 2020, https://www.carbontrust.com/resources/the-eatwell-guide-a-more-sustainable-diet.

Chapter 3

1 **Aune, Dagfinn, et al.** 'Fruit and Vegetable Intake and the Risk of Cardiovascular Disease, Total Cancer and All-Cause Mortality—a Systematic Review and Dose-Response Meta-Analysis of Prospective Studies', *International Journal of Epidemiology*, vol. 46, no. 3, June 2017, pp. 1029–56. academic.oup.com, doi:10.1093/ije/dyw319.

2 **Thomas, D Travis, et al.** 'Position of the Academy of Nutrition and Dietetics, Dietitians of Canada, and the American College of Sports Medicine: Nutrition and Athletic Performance', *Journal of the Academy of Nutrition and Dietetics*, vol. 116, no. 3, March 2016, pp. 501–28. PubMed, doi:10.1016/j.jand.2015.12.006.

3 **Wells, Kimberley R, et al.** 'The Australian Institute of Sport (AIS) and National Eating Disorders Collaboration (NEDC) Position Statement on Disordered Eating in High Performance Sport', *British Journal of Sports Medicine*, July 2020. bjsm.bmj.com, doi:10.1136/bjsports-2019-101813.

4 **Hunt, Janet R, Roughead, Zamzam K.** 'Adaptation of Iron Absorption in Men Consuming Diets with High or Low Iron Bioavailability', *The American Journal of Clinical Nutrition*, vol. 71, no. 1, January 2000, pp. 94–102. academic.oup.com, doi:10.1093/ajcn/71.1.94.

5 **Collings, Rachel, et al.** 'The Absorption of Iron from Whole Diets: A Systematic Review', *The American Journal of Clinical Nutrition*, vol. 98, no. 1, July 2013, pp. 65–81. PubMed, doi:10.3945/ajcn.112.050609.

6 **Melina, Vesanto, et al.** 'Position of the Academy of Nutrition and Dietetics: Vegetarian Diets', *Journal of the Academy of Nutrition and Dietetics*, vol. 116, no. 12, 2016, pp. 1970–80. PubMed, doi:10.1016/j.jand.2016.09.025.

7 **Zhao, Yongdong, et al.** 'Calcium Bioavailability of Calcium Carbonate Fortified Soymilk Is Equivalent to Cow's Milk in Young Women', *The Journal of Nutrition*, vol. 135, no. 10, October 2005, pp. 2379–82. PubMed, doi:10.1093/jn/135.10.2379.

8 **Close, Graeme L, et al.** 'The Effects of Vitamin D3 Supplementation on Serum Total 25[OH]D Concentration and Physical Performance: A Randomised Dose–Response Study', *British Journal of Sports Medicine*, vol. 47, no. 11, July 2013, pp. 692–96. bjsm.bmj.com, doi:10.1136/bjsports-2012-091735.

9 **British Skin Foundation.** 'Sunlight and Vitamin D', https://www.britishskinfoundation.org.uk/sunlight-and-vitamin-d. Accessed September 2020.

10 **The Vegan Society.** "Sources of Vitamin B12', https://www.vegansociety.com/resources/nutrition-and-health/nutrients/vitamin-b12. Accessed February 2021

11 **NHS, UK.** 'Vitamins and Minerals – Vitamin D', 23 October 2017, https://www.nhs.uk/conditions/vitamins-and-minerals/vitamin-d/.

12 **Larson-Meyer, D Enette, et al.** 'Assessment of Nutrient Status in Athletes and the Need for Supplementation', *International Journal of Sport Nutrition and Exercise Metabolism*, vol. 28, no. 2, March 2018, pp. 139–58. journals.humankinetics.com, doi:10.1123/ijsnem.2017-0338.

Chapter 4

1 **Thomas, D Travis, et al.** 'American College of Sports Medicine Joint Position Statement. Nutrition and Athletic Performance', *Medicine and Science in Sports and Exercise*, vol. 48, no. 3, March 2016, pp. 543–68. PubMed, doi:10.1249/MSS.0000000 000000852.

2 **Wolfe, RR, et al.** 'Isotopic Analysis of Leucine and Urea Metabolism in Exercising Humans', *Journal of Applied Physiology: Respiratory, Environmental and Exercise Physiology*, vol. 52, no. 2, February 1982, pp. 458–66. PubMed, doi:10.1152/jappl.1982.52.2.458.

3 **Jäger, Ralf, et al.** 'International Society of Sports Nutrition Position Stand: Protein and Exercise', *Journal of the International Society of Sports Nutrition*, vol. 14, no. 1, June 2017, p. 20. BioMed Central, doi:10.1186/s12970-017-0177-8.

4 **Leidy, Heather J, et al.** 'The Role of Protein in Weight Loss and Maintenance', *The American Journal of Clinical Nutrition*, vol. 101, no. 6, June 2015, pp. 1320S-1329S. academic.oup.com, doi:10.3945/ajcn.114.084038.

5 **Areta, José L, et al.** 'Timing and Distribution of Protein Ingestion during Prolonged Recovery from Resistance Exercise Alters Myofibrillar Protein Synthesis', *The Journal of Physiology*, vol. 591, no. 9, 2013, pp. 2319–31. Wiley Online Library, doi:10.1113/jphysiol.2012.244897.

6 **Macnaughton, Lindsay S, et al.** 'The Response of Muscle Protein Synthesis Following Whole-Body Resistance Exercise Is Greater Following 40 g than 20 g of Ingested Whey Protein', *Physiological Reports*, vol. 4, no. 15, 2016. PubMed, doi:10.14814/phy2.12893.

7 **Moore, Daniel R, et al.** 'Protein Ingestion to Stimulate Myofibrillar Protein Synthesis Requires Greater Relative Protein Intakes in Healthy Older versus Younger Men', *The Journals of Gerontology*, Series A, Biological Sciences and Medical Sciences, vol. 70, no. 1, January 2015, pp. 57–62. PubMed, doi:10.1093/gerona/glu103.

8 **Phillips, Stuart M, et al.** 'Protein 'Requirements' beyond the RDA: Implications for Optimizing Health', *Applied Physiology, Nutrition, and Metabolism*, vol. 41, no. 5, February 2016, pp. 565–72. nrc-prod.literatumonline.com (Atypon), doi:10.1139/apnm-2015-0550.

9 **Aragon, Alan Albert, Schoenfeld, Brad Jon.** 'Nutrient Timing Revisited: Is There a Post-Exercise Anabolic Window?', *Journal of the International Society of Sports Nutrition*, vol. 10, no. 1, January 2013, p. 5. BioMed Central, doi:10.1186/1550-2783-10-5.

10 **Witard, Oliver C, et al.** 'Myofibrillar Muscle Protein Synthesis Rates Subsequent to a Meal in Response to Increasing Doses of Whey Protein at Rest and after Resistance Exercise', *The American Journal of Clinical Nutrition*, vol. 99, no. 1, January 2014, pp. 86–95. PubMed, doi:10.3945/ajcn.112.055517.

11 **Gardner, Christopher D, et al.** 'Maximizing the Intersection of Human Health and the Health of the Environment with Regard to the Amount and Type of Protein Produced and Consumed in the United States', *Nutrition Reviews*, vol. 77, no. 4, April 2019, pp. 197–215. academic.oup.com, doi:10.1093/nutrit/nuy073.

12 **Mariotti, François, Gardner, Christopher D.** 'Dietary Protein and Amino Acids in Vegetarian Diets—A Review', *Nutrients*, vol. 11, no. 11, November 2019, p. 2661. www.mdpi.com, doi:10.3390/nu11112661.

13 **McDougall, John.** 'Plant Foods Have a Complete Amino Acid Composition', *Circulation*, vol. 105, no. 25, June 2002, pp. e197–e197. ahajournals.org (Atypon), doi:10.1161/01.CIR. 000001 8905.97677.1F.

14 **Berrazaga, Insaf, et al.** 'The Role of the Anabolic Properties of Plant- versus Animal-Based Protein Sources in Supporting Muscle Mass Maintenance: A Critical Review', *Nutrients*, vol. 11, no. 8, August 2019. PubMed Central, doi:10.3390/nu11081825.

15 **Young, V R, Pellett, P L.** 'Plant Proteins in Relation to Human Protein and Amino Acid Nutrition', *The American Journal of Clinical Nutrition*, vol. 59, no. 5, May 1994, pp. 1203S-1212S. academic.oup.com, doi:10.1093/ajcn/59.5.1203S.

16 **Rutherfurd, Shane M, et al.** 'Protein Digestibility-Corrected Amino Acid Scores and Digestible Indispensable Amino Acid Scores Differentially Describe Protein Quality in Growing Male Rats', *The Journal of Nutrition*, vol. 145, no. 2, February 2015, pp. 372–79. PubMed, doi:10.3945/jn.114.195438.

17 **Berrazaga, Insaf, et al.** 'The Role of the Anabolic Properties of Plant- versus Animal-Based Protein Sources in Supporting Muscle Mass Maintenance: A Critical Review', *Nutrients*, vol. 11, no. 8, August 2019. PubMed Central, doi:10.3390/nu11081825.

18 **Melina, Vesanto, et al.** 'Position of the Academy of Nutrition and Dietetics: Vegetarian Diets', *Journal of the Academy of Nutrition and Dietetics*, vol. 116, no. 12, 2016, pp. 1970–80. PubMed, doi:10.1016/j.jand.2016.09.025.

19 **Messina, Mark, et al.** 'No Difference Between the Effects of Supplementing With Soy Protein Versus Animal Protein on Gains in Muscle Mass and Strength in Response to Resistance Exercise', *International Journal of Sport Nutrition and Exercise Metabolism*, vol. 28, no. 6, November 2018, pp. 674–85. journals.humankinetics.com, doi:10.1123/ijsnem.2018-0071.

20 **Morton, Robert W, et al.** 'A Systematic Review, Meta-Analysis and Meta-Regression of the Effect of Protein Supplementation on Resistance Training-Induced Gains in Muscle Mass and Strength in Healthy Adults', *British Journal of Sports Medicine*, vol. 52, no. 6, March 2018, pp. 376–84. bjsm.bmj.com, doi:10.1136/bjsports-2017-097608.

21 **Hevia-Larraín, Victoria, et al.** 'High-Protein Plant-Based Diet Versus a Protein-Matched Omnivorous Diet to Support Resistance Training Adaptations: A Comparison Between Habitual Vegans and Omnivores'. Sports Medicine, Feb. 2021. Springer Link, doi:10.1007/s40279-021-01434-9.

22 **Wilkinson, Sarah B, et al.** 'Consumption of Fluid Skim Milk Promotes Greater Muscle Protein Accretion after Resistance Exercise than Does Consumption of an Isonitrogenous and Isoenergetic Soy-Protein Beverage', *The American Journal of Clinical Nutrition*, vol. 85, no. 4, April 2007, pp. 1031–40. PubMed, doi:10.1093/ajcn/85.4.1031.

23 **Phillips, Stuart M, Van Loon, Luc J C.** 'Dietary Protein for Athletes: From Requirements to Optimum Adaptation', *Journal of Sports Sciences*, vol. 29 Suppl 1, 2011, pp. S29-38. PubMed, doi:10.1080/02640414.2011.619204.

24 **van Vliet, Stephan, et al.** 'The Skeletal Muscle Anabolic Response to Plant- versus Animal-Based Protein Consumption', *The Journal of Nutrition*, vol. 145, no. 9, September 2015, pp. 1981–91. academic.oup.com, doi:10.3945/jn.114.204305.

25 **Drummond, Micah J, Rasmussen, Blake B.** 'Leucine-Enriched Nutrients and the Regulation of Mammalian Target of Rapamycin Signalling and Human Skeletal Muscle Protein Synthesis', *Current Opinion in Clinical Nutrition & Metabolic Care*, vol. 11, no. 3, May 2008, pp. 222–226. journals.lww.com, doi:10.1097/MCO.0b013e3282fa17fb.

26 **Burke, Louise M, et al.** 'International Association of Athletics Federations Consensus Statement 2019: Nutrition for Athletics', *International Journal of Sport Nutrition and Exercise Metabolism*, vol. 29, no. 2, March 2019, pp. 73–84. journals.humankinetics.com, doi:10.1123/ijsnem.2019-0065.

Chapter 5

1 **Thomas, D E, et al.** 'Carbohydrate Feeding before Exercise: Effect of Glycemic Index', *International Journal of Sports Medicine*, vol. 12, no. 2, April 1991, pp. 180–86. PubMed, doi:10.1055/s- 2007-1024664.

2 **Thomas, D Travis, et al.** 'Position of the Academy of Nutrition and Dietetics, Dietitians of Canada, and the American College of Sports Medicine: Nutrition and Athletic Performance', *Journal of the Academy of Nutrition and Dietetics*, vol. 116, no. 3, March 2016, pp. 501–28. jandonline.org, doi:10.1016/j.jand.2015.12.006.

3 **Coyle, Edward F.** 'Fluid and Fuel Intake during Exercise', *Journal of Sports Sciences*, vol. 22, no. 1, January 2004, pp. 39–55. tandfonline.com (Atypon), doi:10.1080/0264041031000140545.

4 **Jentjens, Roy L P G, Underwood, Katie et al.** 'Exogenous Carbohydrate Oxidation Rates Are Elevated after Combined Ingestion of Glucose and Fructose during Exercise in the Heat', *Journal of Applied Physiology* (Bethesda, Md.: 1985), vol. 100, no. 3, March 2006, pp. 807–16. PubMed, doi:10.1152/japplphysiol.00322.2005.

5 **Jentjens, Roy L P G, Moseley, Luke et al.** 'Oxidation of Combined Ingestion of Glucose and Fructose during Exercise', *Journal of Applied Physiology* (Bethesda, Md.: 1985), vol. 96, no. 4, April 2004, pp. 1277–84. PubMed, doi:10.1152/japplphysiol.00974.2003.

6 **Shirreffs, Susan M, Sawka, Michael N.** 'Fluid and Electrolyte Needs for Training, Competition, and Recovery', *Journal of Sports Sciences*, vol. 29 Suppl 1, 2011, pp. S39-46. PubMed, doi:10.1080/02640414.2011.614269.

7 **Hew-Butler, Tamara, et al.** 'Updated Fluid Recommendation: Position Statement from the International Marathon Medical Directors Association (IMMDA)', *Clinical Journal of Sport Medicine: Official Journal of the Canadian Academy of Sport Medicine*, vol. 16, no. 4, July 2006, pp. 283–92. PubMed, doi:10.1097/00042752-200607000-00001.

8 **Noakes, Tim, IMMDA.** 'Fluid Replacement during Marathon Running', *Clinical Journal of Sport Medicine: Official Journal of the Canadian Academy of Sport Medicine*, vol. 13, no. 5, September 2003, pp. 309–18.

9 **Schoenfeld, Brad Jon, et al.** 'The Effect of Protein Timing on Muscle Strength and Hypertrophy: A Meta-Analysis', *Journal of the International Society of Sports Nutrition*, vol. 10, no. 1, December 2013, p. 53. BioMed Central, doi:10.1186/1550-2783-10-53. PubMed, doi:10.1097/00042752-200309000-00007.

10 **Jäger, Ralf, et al.** 'International Society of Sports Nutrition Position Stand: Protein and Exercise', *Journal of the International Society of Sports Nutrition*, vol. 14, no. 1, June 2017, p. 20. BioMed Central, doi:10.1186/s12970-017-0177-8.

11 **Moore, Daniel R, et al.** 'Ingested Protein Dose Response of Muscle and Albumin Protein Synthesis after Resistance Exercise in Young Men', *The American Journal of Clinical Nutrition*, vol. 89, no. 1, January 2009, pp. 161–68. *PubMed*, doi:10.3945/ajcn.2008.26401.

12 **Burke, Louise M, Hawley, John A.** 'Effects of Short-Term Fat Adaptation on Metabolism and Performance of Prolonged Exercise', *Medicine and Science in Sports and Exercise*, vol. 34, no. 9, September 2002, pp. 1492–98. PubMed, doi:10.1097/00005768-200209000-00015.

13 **Stellingwerff, Trent, et al.** 'Decreased PDH Activation and Glycogenolysis during Exercise Following Fat Adaptation with Carbohydrate Restoration', *American Journal of Physiology, Endocrinology and Metabolism*, vol. 290, no. 2, February 2006, pp. E380-388. PubMed, doi: 10.1152/ajpendo.00268.2005.

14 **Burke, Louise M, Sharma, Avish P et al.** 'Crisis of Confidence Averted: Impairment of Exercise Economy and Performance in Elite Race Walkers by Ketogenic Low Carbohydrate, High Fat (LCHF) Diet Is Reproducible', *PLOS One*, vol. 15, no. 6, June 2020, p. e0234027. PLoS Journals, doi:10.1371/journal.pone.0234027.

15 **Burke, Louise M, Ross, Megan L, et al.** 'Low Carbohydrate, High Fat Diet Impairs Exercise Economy and Negates the Performance Benefit from Intensified Training in Elite Race Walkers', *The Journal of Physiology*, vol. 595, no. 9, May 2017, pp. 2785–807. PubMed Central, doi:10.1113/JP273230.

16 **Marquet, Laurie-Anne, et al.** 'Periodization of Carbohydrate Intake: Short-Term Effect on Performance', *Nutrients*, vol. 8, no. 12, November 2016. PubMed, doi:10.3390/nu8120755.

17 **Aird, T P, et al.** 'Effects of Fasted vs Fed-State Exercise on Performance and Post-Exercise Metabolism: A Systematic Review and Meta-Analysis', *Scandinavian Journal of Medicine & Science in Sports*, vol. 28, no. 5, May 2018, pp. 1476–93. PubMed, doi:10.1111/sms.13054.

18 **Terada, Tasuku, et al.** 'Overnight Fasting Compromises Exercise Intensity and Volume during Sprint Interval Training but Improves High-Intensity Aerobic Endurance', *The Journal of Sports Medicine and Physical Fitness*, vol. 59, no. 3, March 2019, pp. 357–65. PubMed, doi:10.23736/S0022-4707.18.08281-6.

Chapter 6

1 **Maughan, Ronald J, et al.** 'IOC Consensus Statement: Dietary Supplements and the High-Performance Athlete', *British Journal of Sports Medicine*, vol. 52, no. 7, April 2018, pp. 439–55. bjsm.bmj.com, doi:10.1136/bjsports-2018-099027.

Chapter 8

1 **Public Health England.** 'Government Dietary Recommendations', 2016 https://assets.publishing.service.gov.uk/government/uploads/system/uploads/attachment_data/file/618167/government_dietary_recommendations.pdf Accessed February 2021.

2 **European Commission.** 'Additives' https://ec.europa.eu/food/safety/food_improvement_agents/additives_en Accessed February 2021

3 **Laudisi, Federica, et al.** 'Impact of Food Additives on Gut Homeostasis.' *Nutrients*, vol. 11, no. 10, Oct. 2019. *PubMed Central*, doi:10.3390/nu11102334.

4 **Library of Congress.** 'European Union: "Milk" Cannot Be Used to Market Purely Plant-Based Products' https://www.loc.gov/law/foreign-news/article/european-union-milk-cannot-be-used-to-market-purely-plant-based-products/#:%7E:text=(June%2027%2C%202017)%20On,(e.g.%2C%20tofu%20butter). Accessed February 2021

5 **Lin, Lin, et al.** 'Evidence of Health Benefits of Canola Oil.' *Nutrition Reviews*, vol. 71, no. 6, June 2013, pp. 370–85. *PubMed Central*, doi:10.1111/nure.12033.

Resources

www.vegansociety.com The website of the UK Vegan Society provides comprehensive resources on the vegan lifestyle, nutrition, health and the environment, as well as tasty recipes.

www.vegsoc.org The website of the UK Vegetarian Society provides clear information and downloadable resources on health and nutrition, animal welfare, sustainability, the environment and recipes.

www.vivahealth.org.uk The website of the charity Viva! Health provides information, articles and downloadable resources on vegan nutrition and health topics.

www.veganhealth.org is a US website providing a comprehensive set of resources on vegan nutrition, including research summaries, nutrition and health articles, and meal plans.

www.health4performance.co.uk Sponsored by the British Association of Sport and Exercise Medicine, this website provides information on and practical help for Relative Energy Deficiency in Sport (RED-S).

www.sportsdietitians.com.au The website of Sports Dietitians Australia provides nutrition information and advice for different sports and factsheets covering a wide range of sports nutrition topics.

www.bda.co.uk The website of the British Dietetic Association provides downloadable fact sheets on a wide range of nutrition topics.

www.eatright.org The website of the US Academy of Nutrition and Dietetics provides articles and videos on a range of food, health and fitness topics.

www.nomeatathlete.com This US website provides articles and resources on vegan nutrition and fitness.

www.meatfreemondays.com is a not-for-profit campaign launched by Paul, Mary and Stella McCartney. The website includes news, advice and vegan recipes.

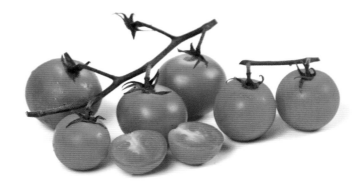

Metric/Imperial Conversion Chart

WEIGHTS

Metric	Imperial
15 g	½ oz
25 g	1 oz
40 g	1½ oz
50 g	2 oz
75 g	3 oz
100 g	3½ oz
125 g	4 oz
150 g	5 oz
175 g	6 oz
200 g	7 oz
225 g	8 oz
250 g	9 oz
275 g	10 oz
300 g	11 oz
350 g	12 oz
375 g	13 oz
400 g	14 oz
425 g	15 oz
450 g	1 lb
500 g	1 lb 2 oz
1 kg	2¼ lb

VOLUMES

Metric	Imperial	US cups
5 ml		1 teaspoon
15 ml	½ fl oz	1 tablespoon
25 ml	1 fl oz	⅛ cup
50 ml	2 fl oz	¼ cup
75 ml	3 fl oz	⅓ cup
125 ml	4 fl oz	½ cup
150 ml	5 fl oz/¼ pint	⅔ cup
175 ml	6 fl oz	¾ cup
200 ml	7 fl oz	⅞ cup
250 ml	8 fl oz	1 cup
300 ml	½ pint	1¼ cups
500 ml	18 fl oz	2 cups
600 ml	1 pint	2¼ cups
1 litre	1¾ pints	4 cups

All equivalents are rounded
for practical convenience

US CUP TO GRAM CONVERSIONS OF COMMON INGREDIENTS

1 cup flour	125 g
1 cup rolled oats	85 g
1 cup sugar	200 g
1 cup large dried pulses (e.g. chickpeas)	170 g
1 cup small dried pulses (e.g. lentils)	200 g
1 cup rice	200 g
1 cup nuts	125 g
1 cup seeds	160 g
1 cup non-dairy spread	225 g

OVEN TEMPERATURES

Celsius	Fahrenheit
140	275
150	300
160	325
180	350
190	375
200	400
220	425

Index

super-seedy bars 198
supplements, dietary 11, 25, 26, 29–30, 37, 49
sweet potato, beetroot and chickpea salad 104
syrups 55, 58

T

tabbouleh 87
tagine, chickpea and butternut squash 116
tahini 61
tart, raspberry semi-freddo 164
tempeh 61
Teriyaki tempeh noodle bowl 105
Thai green curry with crispy tofu balls 133
three-bean chilli with cashew cream 134
three-nut butter 193
toasting nuts and seeds 57
tofu 61
tofu satay skewers 151
tofu scramble 80
tomato and coconut dal with crispy tofu and cashews 137
type 2 diabetes 14, 15, 19

V

vanilla and cinnamon quinoa porridge 77
Vegan Athlete's Plate 6, 21–2
    adjustments for levels of training 23, 24, 40–7
    food groups 22–3
vegan diet
    avoiding nutrition pit falls 24–9
    best way to get protein 33

defined 6
environmental impact 20
food swops 50–1
growing popularity 6–7
health advantage 14–16
how to adopt a 50–1
nutrient levels 16
nutritional myths 11–13
overly restrictive 7, 10
performance advantage 16–18
popular ingredients 55–61
prejudice against 10
vegetarian diet 14, 15–16, 17, 50
vitamin B6 25
Vitamin B12 24, 25–6, 29, 30
vitamin C 12, 18, 26–7, 30
vitamin D 28–9, 30–1
vitamin E 18
vitamin K 17

W

weight loss 7, 12, 47
weight management 15, 19, 32, 44

Y

yeast, nutritional 59
yogurt alternative 28
yogurt pot, fruit and granola 74
yogurt, strawberry frozen 161

Z

zinc 22, 24, 29